THE COMPLETE
Keto Diet
BOOK 2021

The Keto Diet Cookbook with Quick and Healthy Recipes incl. 5 Week Weight Loss Plan

JOHN C. SMITH

Table of Contents

Dinner Recipes 74

INTRODUCTION

The Ketogenic Diet is a high fat diet which appears to benefit some people with epilepsy, especially children. It is not a magic cure but one alternative to the various anti-epileptic medications currently available. The ketogenic diet offers the advantage of improved seizure control for some children, and in some cases, improved mental alertness with fewer medications.

The ketogenic diet is often regarded as a difficult regimen to follow, however, with practice, and an understanding what the diet aims to achieve, it can be reduced to a manageable routine. The basic aim is to switch the body's primary fuel source from carbohydrates (like bread and sugar)to fats. This is done by increasing the intake of fats and greatly reducing the intake of carbohydrates. The real difficulty is that the diet is so restrictive, that all foods eaten must be weighed out to a tenth of a gram during meal preparation, and a participant may not eat anything which is not "prescribed" by the dietician. The level of carbohydrates allowed is very low so that even the small amount of sugar in most liquid or chewable medications will prevent the diet from working.

As examples, a typical meal might include some type of meat with green vegetables cooked with a mayonnaise sauce or a lot of butter. Heavy cream may be included on the side for drinking. Another meal might consist of bacon and eggs with a lot of butter or oil added, and heavy cream to drink. A very high ratio of fats to carbohydrates must be maintained with a low total calorie intake for the diet to be successful.

What is a Keto Diet?

A keto diet is well-known for being a low carb diet, in which the body produces ketones in the liver to be used as energy. It's referred to by many different names – ketogenic diet, low carb diet, low carb high fat (LCHF), and so on. Though some of these other "names" have different standards, we'll stick with the standards of keto.

When you eat something high in carbs, your body will produce glucose and insulin. Glucose is the easiest molecule for your body to convert and use as energy, so it will be chosen over any other energy source.

Insulin is produced to process the glucose in your bloodstream, by taking it around the body. Since the glucose is being used as a primary energy, your fats are not needed and are therefore stored. Typically on a normal, higher carbohydrate diet, the body will use glucose as the main form of energy.

By lowering the intake of carbs, the body is induced into a state known as ketosis.

What is Ketosis?

Ketosis is an everyday process of the body, regardless of the number of carbs you eat. Your body can adapt very well, processing different types of nutrients into the fuels that it needs. Proteins, fats, and carbs can all be processed for use. Eating a low carb, high fat diet just ramps up this process, which is a normal and safe chemical reaction.

When you eat carbohydrate-based foods or excess amounts of protein, your body will break this down into sugar – known as glucose. Why? Glucose is needed in the creation of ATP (an energy mole-cule), which is a fuel that is needed for the daily activities and maintenance inside our bodies.

If you've ever used a calculator to determine your caloric needs, you will see that your body uses up quite a lot of calories. It's true, our bodies use up much of the nutrients we intake just to maintain itself on a daily basis. If you eat enough food, there will likely be excess glucose your body doesn't need.

There are two main things that happen to glucose if your body doesn't need it:

- Glycogenesis. Excess glucose will be converted to glycogen, and stored in your liver and muscles. Estimates show that only about half of your daily energy can be stored as glycogen.
- Lipogenesis. If there's already enough glycogen in your muscles and liver, any extra glucose will be converted into fats and stored.

So, what happens to you once your body has no more glucose or glycogen? Ketosis happens.

When your body has no access to food, like when you are sleeping, the body will burn fat and create molecules called ketones. This is what happens on a ketogenic diet - we burn fat for energy. We can thank our body's ability to switch metabolic pathways for that.

These ketones (acetoacetate) are created when the body breaks down fats, creating fatty acids, and burned off in the liver in a process called beta-oxidation. The end result of this process is the creation of 2 other ketones (BHB and acetone), which are used as fuel by the muscles and brain.

Although glucose is the main source of fuel for most people, these fatty acids (BHB and acetone) are used by the brain cells when carbohydrate or food intake is low. In simpler terms, since you have no more glucose or glycogen, ketosis kicks in and your body will use your stored/consumed fat as energy.

Ketosis is pretty amazing, and in fact, gets even better. Studies show that the body and brain actually prefer using ketones, being able to run 70% more efficiently than glucose. From an evolutionary standpoint, this makes perfect sense.

What are benefit of Keto Diet?

1) **A keto diet leads to weight loss:** When you avoid carbohydrates, your body starts burning stored fat; it will automatically cause decreased appetite. On the other hand, you will experience higher energy levels.

2) **Mental clarity and better concentration:** On a keto diet, our brain uses ketones as the main fuel; consequently, it reduces the levels of toxins. It will significantly improve your cognitive functions, mental focus, concentration, and mental performance.

3) **Health benefits:** A keto diet restricts carbohydrates; they can be found in unhealthy sugary foods, refined grains such as bread, pasta and white rice. On the other hand, it promotes foods that are loaded with high-quality protein (it is essential for building muscle), good fat, and healthy veggies. Many studies have proven that low-carb diets can significantly improve health. They measured the main outcomes such as LDL cholesterol, HDL cholesterol, blood sugar levels, triglycerides, and weight loss.

Fatty fish such (for example, tuna and salmon) is well known for its ability to lower triglycerides; consequently, it can reduce the risk of stroke. Unsaturated fat-packed foods such as seeds, nuts and unrefined vegetable oils can help your body to lower triglycerides, too. In addition, cutting out carbs can reduce insulin levels and regulate blood sugar. Not only can keto diets improve your physical performance and boost weight loss, but they also treat some serious conditions. Keto diets have proven beneficial in treating several brain disorders such as epilepsy in children. Moreover, ketogenic diets are incredibly effective in treating metabolic syndrome.

How to start keto Diet?

Five Steps to Starting a Successful Keto Diet

Now that you know the what and the why behind the ketogenic diet, let's learn about how you can get started. Although there are many different approaches to keto you can try, most of your results will come from following these steps:

Step 1: Determine Your Fitness Goal

Before going into any diet, the first step should always be identifying your "why" or your primary goal - this will establish your dietary needs and guide your focus moving forward. As well as how you can determine if your hard work is paying off.

There are four main reasons why someone would consider changing up their eating, and not all of them are a great fit for keto:

- Weight loss
- Muscle Gain
- Improved Performance
- Improved Health

Weight Loss

Weight loss or fat loss is the most common reason why someone would consider trying keto. If this is your goal, maintaining a calorie deficit is your number one agenda. And your progress can be measured by seeing the number on the scale decrease or by adjusting your body composition, which can be assessed using any body fat analysis tool.

Muscle Gain

Muscle gain is essentially weight gain and is not always the ideal starting place for everyone. Moreover, a ketogenic diet may not be the best diet for building muscle, given the beneficial role of carbohydrates in training, and muscle recovery. But that doesn't stop everyone, and some people will see results. Achieving more muscle will require you to focus on extra calories, training and macronutrient balance. And to accurately measure your progress, a body composition test is required.

Improved Performance

Fat can be an abundant and valuable source of energy that many athletes would like to tap into. This is precisely why keto is also used to increase performance in endurance athletes and those who do not require consistent explosive power or frequent high-intensity training. Nutrient timing and adequate fueling is the primary focus of this goal, and performance progress can be measured through fitness goals or assessing metabolic efficiency.

Improved Health

Improving health is not always a primary goal of keto dieters - unless health is improved as a result of losing weight. This is because a keto diet is fairly restrictive, and getting high amounts of vitamins and minerals (micronutrients) can be challenging. If you are looking to keto to improve your nutrition, nutritious food choices should be top of mind. Progress towards this goal can be measured through biometric testing (health assessments).

Step 2: Calculate Your Daily Calorie Goal

Once you've identified your main health and fitness goal, the next step is to calculate how many calories you need to eat a day in order to lose weight, gain weight, or maintain your weight. The easiest way to do this is with an online calorie calculator or by downloading a fitness app that uses your age, height, weight, gender, and fitness level to estimate your daily needs.

Step 3: Calculate Your Keto Macros

While it is your calorie control that has the largest impact on your weight, understanding your keto macros is still pretty fundamental to your success. Especially if you are trying to get into ketosis, hitting your carb goal each day is crucial.

The keto diet is designed to follow strict macronutrient targets, including high fat and extremely low carb intake. For most people, this breakdown looks something like the following:

- 70% of calories from fat
- 25% of calories from protein
- 5% of calories from carbs

However, the exact ideal macro ratio for you can be dependent on your fitness, metabolic efficiency, and other individual considerations. To calculate your personal keto macro you can use any online or offline keto macro calculator.

Step 4: Plan Your Keto Menu

Now you're ready to start planning your dream keto menu. But before you start loading up on bacon and cheese, there are a few things to consider when it comes to your food choices. The nutrition and quality of the foods you eat are still important for your overall health and wellbeing. Additionally, choosing more nutritious foods may help with energy levels, mood, and potentially cravings - helping you stick to your ketogenic diet longer.

What to Eat on a Keto Diet

Keto emphasizes higher fat intake and little carb intake. This can make meal planning challenging since a large number of high carb foods are not considered keto-friendly - like grains, breads, starchy veggies, and fruits.

Additionally, carbs tend to be the bulk of most people's diets - meaning you have to find a keto alternative or change the way you think about meals in general. Some of the best staples for any keto diet should include healthy carb substitutes. Many veggies work great for this, like:

- Cauliflower rice
- Mashed cauliflower
- Portobello mushroom "buns"
- Spaghetti squash
- Zucchini noodles (or "zoodles")
- Lettuce wraps

Help keep your nutrition in check, have the bulk of your keto diet should consist of nutrient-rich low carb veggies, quality proteins, and healthy fats to ensure you are getting the right balance and overall good nutrition to keep you going.

Keto Food List

Here is a brief overview of what you should and shouldn't eat on the keto diet:

Do Not Eat

- Grains – wheat, corn, rice, cereal, etc.
- Sugar – honey, agave, maple syrup, etc.
- Fruit – apples, bananas, oranges, etc.
- Tubers – potato, yams, etc.

Do Eat

- Meats – fish, beef, lamb, poultry, eggs, etc.
- Low-carb vegetables – spinach, kale, broccoli, and other low carb veggies.
- High-fat dairy – hard cheeses, high fat cream, butter, etc.
- Nuts and seeds – macadamias, walnuts, sunflower seeds, etc.
- Avocado and berries – raspberries, blackberries, and other low glycemic impact berries
- Sweeteners – stevia, erythritol, monk fruit, and other low-carb sweeteners.

- Other fats – coconut oil, high-fat salad dressing, saturated fats, etc.

Step 5: Stick to Your Keto Goals

Planning a keto menu is only half the battle; your progress is the result of consistency. Meaning, you've got to stick to your diet plan for more than a few weeks. But sticking to your diet is not based on sheer willpower, as much as it is developing healthy habits and routines that allow you to be successful. This includes making healthy decisions easier and adding some friction to less healthy habits. It also isn't required for you to be perfect on your keto diet for it to be effective. It is possible to have a keto cheat day or go off course and still see progress. As long as you stick to your calorie goals consistently, and keep working at it.

How to weight loss more effectively with Keto diet?

Once you've made it through the first week of keto and you are in ketosis, fat will steadily fall off your body (as long as you are in a calorie deficit). The average weight loss at this point is around 1-2 pounds per week — the majority of it coming from fat. As you get closer to your goal weight and your overall body weight decreases, weight loss will slow down. This happens because as your weight decreases so will your daily caloric needs. For this reason, you may want to recalculate your calorie needs every month or so. Keep in mind that weight loss may not be consistent either. You might have some weeks where it seems you haven't lost anything — then you'll weigh yourself a week or two later and be down 3-4 pounds. What is behind the seemingly unpredictable and unique nature of your weight loss rate? Here are some of the critical factors that determine how fast the pounds will come off:

Your calorie deficit: The one factor that leads to the most significant and consistent weight loss is a calorie deficit. In other words, when we consume fewer calories than we need to maintain our weight, we will lose weight. This means that your weight loss rate will usually increase as your total calorie consumption decreases. However, there are limits to how far you should take you should take your deficit. The human body is designed to prevent massive amounts of weight loss during times of starvation via mechanisms that make long-term fat loss much harder to achieve and maintain. Because of this, it is never a good idea to starve yourself for extended periods of time. Research indicates that calorie deficits above 30% are enough to stimulate some of these counterproductive mechanisms for long-term fat loss.

Your current health status: Your overall health plays a major role in how fast you will lose weight and adapt to a lower carb diet. If you have any hormonal or metabolic issues, weight loss might be slower or a bit more challenging than expected. Insulin resistance, excess visceral fat, and thyroid issues, for example, can all have a significant impact on your weight loss rate.

Your body composition: Do you have a lot of fat to lose? How much muscle do you have? The people who have the most to lose will tend to shred the fat at a much faster rate than those who have a few extra pounds to burn off. This phenomenon is mostly explained by the fact that obese individuals can easily maintain a much larger calorie deficit, which will result in faster weight loss. Muscle mass also plays a vital role in weight loss because it helps keep your metabolic rate from dropping significantly as you lose weight. This can help stabilize your weight loss rate and may even prevent a dreaded weight loss plateau.

Your daily habits: Your daily habits will make or break your weight loss efforts. Consistency is the key to keto success. Are you eating clean keto foods or high-fat junk foods with low-quality ingredients? Are you watching out for hidden carbs? Are you exercising? Eating the right foods in the right amounts for your goals and adding more physical activity to your daily life are the most important pieces of a smooth and successful body transformation. When we take a step back and look at the bigger picture of our fat loss rate, predictable patterns began to emerge. For example, the people who typically see the slowest weight loss are those who are sedentary and overweight with poor metabolic health and eating habits that don't exercise or keep track of their carb and/or calorie consumption.

Conversely, those who start with more muscle and decent metabolic health that are disciplined enough to stick to their diet plan, maintain a calorie deficit, and increase their physical activity levels will typically lose weight more quickly and get the results they want. In general, everyone's health and lifestyle is different, which means the weight loss rate for each person is going to be different too. We do, however, share one thing in common: each one of us can optimize our body composition with our diets.

How to Avoid Muscle Loss on Keto?

The most important macronutrient for preserving and building lean muscle is protein. Carbs help preserve muscle mass to some extent, but protein is — without a doubt — the most important macronutrient that you must eat enough if you don't want to lose muscle.

Protein consumption is especially crucial on the ketogenic diet. Without dietary carbs to provoke an anabolic (muscle building) response, you will tend to lose muscle more rapidly without adequate protein intake on keto. With that being said, research has also found that ketones have a muscle preserving effect. Because of this, it is reasonable to suggest that you should eat just enough protein to maintain muscle mass without eating so much protein that you decrease your ketone levels.

The most common ketogenic diet FAQs and answer

Many people have questions about the ketogenic diet before they get started. So, we've compiled a list of answers to the frequently asked questions that people have.

What is keto-adaptation and what does it feel like?

The term keto-adaptation refers to your body's transition from burning primarily glucose as fuel, to being able to also use ketones produced from burning body fat.It will take a few days or weeks to feel your absolute best on keto. You may experience symptoms of carbohydrate withdrawal at first, but once you become fat-adapted, you'll find that you won't crave carbs as much anymore.

What is the "keto flu" and how can I avoid it?

Your body has always relied on glucose as its primary source of energy. Therefore, when you cut carbohydrates drastically, the body is essentially freaking out, until it eventually switches its metabolism to burning fat. This period of adaptation causes the mild physical weakness or lack of energy typical of the flu. This state is temporary and the transition can be facilitated by a few preventive measures, such as keeping hydrated and having enough salt. Visit our keto side effects page to know more about effective ways to help circumvent the keto flu.

How long does it take to become keto-adapted?

Most research papers and anecdotal evidence you'll come across state that keto-adaptation can last up to four weeks. The more determined you are to avoid carbs in the first weeks of a ketogenic diet, the quicker you'll be over the hump on your keto-adaptation. You can also hasten it by engaging in any form of sustained physical activity which will force your body to tap into its fat stores.

What does be in a state of ketosis mean?

Being in a state of ketosis means that your body, more precisely your liver, is producing higher levels of ketone bodies to supply energy for your brain, heart and muscles. For that to happen, carbohydrates need to be sufficiently restricted and your protein intake capped at a certain level – which is explained in our protein and keto page. A state of ketosis can come and go through any day but with time you'll learn how to stay ketotic for longer.

How can I tell if I am in ketosis?

There are a few telltale signs that you are in ketosis. If you wake up with a fruity, metallic taste in your mouth, also called keto breath, it is an indication that your body is effectively manufacturing ketones. You could also experience a certain mental sharpness when the body runs high on ketones. For those looking to be more sure of whether ketosis is taking place, you can use home tests such as blood tests, urine tests or a breathalyzer to test your level of ketosis.

What may put me out of ketosis and how can I get back into it quickly?

It is easy to get out of ketosis. It will usually happen immediately after meals, even if they contain a small to medium amounts of carbs, and can last for up to a few hours. This is normal, your body will always choose to revert back to glucose if some is available.

We don't recommend hacking ketosis with keto esters (essentially artificial ketones you ingest), as they are not fully clinically tested yet. However, there are a few things that can help promote a state of ketosis. These include incorporating periods of fasting or consuming certain types of fat that are very ketogenic, like MCTs.

Should I track my ketones levels? If yes, how?

There are a few ways that you can track your ketone levels, depending mainly on your budget. Urine ketone strips are the easiest to come by and they are relatively cheap, which enables you to test more often. However, they only give you an estimation of the range of your ketone levels. If you want to gain a bit more insights about how your body is handling your ketogenic diet, you may want to check out our guide to measuring ketones on a ketogenic diet.

Will the diet help with weight loss and improve my sugar levels?

Two of the main benefits of the ketogenic diet is its effect in helping people to lose weight and lowering blood glucose levels. If you take medication that can cause hypos, such as insulin, sulphonylureas or glinides, you will need to take care to avoid hypos occurring. Speak to your doctor who will be able to advise you on what precautions to take to reduce the risk of hypos occurring.

Do I need to count or restrict calories?

No, although there is a subset of ketogenic diets, known as a calorie-restricted ketogenic diet, which is specifically restricted in calories. If and when followed correctly though, a ketogenic diet can be eaten to satiety. This is, in part, because the diet does not usually promote weight gain, as it lowers levels of the fat storage hormone insulin.

What does insulin load and glycemic index refer to?

Different foods will influence insulin levels differently, this is known as the insulin load of a food. The glycemic index (GI) tells you how slowly or quickly that food is likely to increase blood glucose levels. On a ketogenic diet, you'll want to avoid high GI foods as they will not support ketosis. You can visit our page on which foods to eat on a ketogenic diet to learn more about this.

I'm physically active, can I still do a ketogenic diet?

Many people are concerned that a ketogenic diet might not be compatible with a high-energy lifestyle. Research actually suggests the opposite, in that ketones can improve performance. However, you should reduce your workout intensity or not engage in anything that demands a ton of glucose while you try to get fat-adapted. You can read about this subject in our page about exercise on a ketogenic diet.

Do I need to incorporate carbohydrate re-feed days?

Different types of ketogenic diets exist, some of them giving the flexibility to live a slightly more sane life with carb re-feed days. These can be helpful as an induction phase to a ketogenic diet, for active people who might need carbs around the time of their workout, or to accommodate social circumstances. You can visit our page on the types of ketogenic diets to decide which one is best or right for you.

What is the difference between a low-carbohydrate diet and a ketogenic diet?

Ketogenic diets are a slightly more extreme form of low carbohydrate diets. While up to 150 grams of carbohydrates a day may be regarded as low carb, entering a state of ketosis usually requires lowering carbohydrates to a level of under 50 grams a day. A ketogenic diet is also a lot higher in fat and lower in protein.

Can I practice intermittent fasting on keto?

Yes, you can. It is a very useful tool to boost ketone levels and fat burning. However, you should get keto-adapted first before attempting it.

If you are on diabetes medication that can cause hypos, it is important to check which precautions to take before adding intermittent fasting to a ketogenic diet.

Tips Before Starting

Some people don't believe in counting calories on a ketogenic diet, but I am one of the few that does. For most normal people, the amounts of fats and protein will be enough to naturally keep you satia-ted and naturally keep you in a calorie deficit. Though, the average American is not always normal.

There's tons of hormone, endocrine, and deficiency problems that we need to take into account. That said, it doesn't always allow you to lose weight when you are consuming more than your own body is expending. "Macros" is a shortened version of macronutrients. These are the "big 3" – fats, proteins, and carbs. You can use a calculator to find out how much or how little of each you need in order to attain your goals.

A lot of people take their macros as a "set in stone" type of thing. You shouldn't worry about hitting the mark every single day to the dot. If you're a few calories over some days, a few calories under on others – it's fine. Everything will even itself out in the end. It's all about a long-term plan that can work for you, and not the other way around.

I wanted to put it out there that I made this meal plan specifically with women in mind. I took an average of about 150 women and what their macros were. The end result was 1600 calories – broken down into 136g of fat, 74g of protein, and 20g net carbs a day. This is all built around a sedentary lifestyle, like most of us live. If you need to increase or decrease calories, you will need to do that on your own terms.

To increase calories, it's quite easy – increase the amounts of fat you eat. Olive oil, coconut oil, ma-cadamia nuts, and butter are great ways to increase fats without getting too much of the other stuff in the way. Drizzle it on salads, slather it on vegetables, snack on it, do what you need to do to make it work in your favor!

To decrease calories, you will have to think about what you need. Most likely, you will need less pro-tein as well. So, keep in mind the portions of sizes of meals. Decrease them as you need to, or see fit. Last, but certainly not least, is sticking to the diet! Ketosis is a process that happens in your body. You can't just have "that one" cheat meal. If you do, it can hamper progress for up to a week before your body is back in ketosis and normally functioning again.

You want to keep your cheats to none. Be prepared, make sure you're eating what you need to be satiated ("full"), and make sure you're satisfied with what you're eating. If you have to force yourself to eat something, it will never work out in the end. This is just a guideline on how you can eat on a ketogenic diet, so you're very welcome to change up what kind of foods you eat!

35-Days Keto Diet Weight Loss Challenge

First Week Meal Plan

Day	Breakfast	Lunch	Dinner
Sunday	Cheese Omelette (Page No. 26)	Chewy Coconut Chunks (Page No. 52)	Chicken and Snap (Page No. 78)
Monday	Butter Coffee (Page No. 25)	Low Carb Smoothie (Page No. 50)	Keto chicken casserole (Page No. 78)
Tuesday	Low Carb Keto Coffee Recipe (Page No. 25)	Peanut Butter Biscuits (Page No. 52)	Keto chicken enchilada bowl (Page No. 77)
Wednesday	Butter Coffee (Page No. 25)	Creamy Tuscan Garlic Chicken (Page No. 51)	Chicken salad with guacamole (Page No. 80)
Thursday	Egg Medley Muffins (Page No. 27)	Keto Avocado Smoothie (Page No. 51)	Fried Chicken Recipe (Page No. 74)
Friday	Low Carb Keto Coffee Recipe (Page No. 25)	Green Keto Smoothie (Page No. 50)	Keto chicken enchilada bowl (Page No. 77)
Saturday	Keto Coffee Recipe (Page No. 25)	Charming Keto Carrot Cake (Page No. 53)	Fried Chicken Recipe (Page No. 74)

35-Days Keto Diet Weight Loss Challenge

Second Week Meal Plan

Day	Breakfast	Lunch	Dinner
Sunday	Egg Medley Muffins (Page No. 27)	Low Carb Smoothie (Page No. 50)	Fried Chicken Recipe (Page No. 74)
Monday	Low Carb Keto Coffee Recipe (Page No. 25)	Green Keto Smoothie (Page No. 50)	Baked Eggs and Zoodles (Page No. 74)
Tuesday	Keto Coffee Recipe (Page No. 25)	Almond & Vanilla Keto Cheesecake (Page No. 53)	Keto pizza chaffles (Page No. 88)
Wednesday	Coffee Egg Latte (Page No. 26)	Charming Keto Carrot Cake (Page No. 53)	Keto chicken enchilada bowl (Page No. 77)
Thursday	Butter Coffee (Page No. 25)	Keto Avocado Smoothie (Page No. 51)	Chicken salad with guacamole (Page No. 80)
Friday	Keto Coffee Recipe (Page No. 25)	Chewy Coconut Chunks (Page No. 52)	Chicken and Snap (Page No. 78)
Saturday	Low Carb Keto Coffee Recipe (Page No. 25)	Green Keto Smoothie (Page No. 50)	Fried Chicken Recipe (Page No. 74)

35-Days Keto Diet Weight Loss Challenge

Third Week Meal Plan

Day	Breakfast	Lunch	Dinner
Sunday	Egg Medley Muffins (Page No. 27)	Green Keto Smoothie (Page No. 50)	Baked Eggs and Zoodles (Page No. 74)
Monday	Butter Coffee (Page No. 25)	Charming Keto Carrot Cake (Page No. 53)	Chicken salad with guacamole (Page No. 80)
Tuesday	Coffee Egg Latte (Page No. 26)	Chewy Coconut Chunks (Page No. 52)	Fried Chicken Recipe (Page No. 74)
Wednesday	Butter Coffee (Page No. 25)	Green Keto Smoothie (Page No. 50)	Chicken and Snap (Page No. 78)
Thursday	Keto Coffee Recipe (Page No. 25)	Peanut Butter Biscuits (Page No. 52)	Keto chicken casserole (Page No. 78)
Friday	Butter Coffee (Page No. 25)	Low Carb Smoothie (Page No. 50)	Fried Chicken Recipe (Page No. 74)
Saturday	Keto Coffee Recipe (Page No. 25)	Almond & Vanilla Keto Cheesecake (Page No. 53)	Keto pizza chaffles (Page No. 88)

35-Days Keto Diet Weight Loss Challenge

Fourth Week Meal Plan

Day	Breakfast	Lunch	Dinner
Sunday	Butter Coffee (Page No. 25)	Green Keto Smoothie (Page No. 50)	Keto chicken enchilada bowl (Page No. 77)
Monday	Cheese Omelette (Page No. 26)	Keto Avocado Smoothie (Page No. 51)	Keto chicken casserole (Page No. 78)
Tuesday	Low Carb Keto Coffee Recipe (Page No. 25)	Peanut Butter Biscuits (Page No. 52)	Fried eggs with kale (Page No. 93)
Wednesday	Cheese Omelette (Page No. 26)	Creamy Tuscan Garlic Chicken (Page No. 51)	Scrambled Eggs with Basil and Butter (Page No. 92)
Thursday	Coffee Egg Latte (Page No. 26)	Green Keto Smoothie (Page No. 50)	Baked Eggs and Zoodles (Page No. 74)
Friday	Cheese Omelette (Page No. 26)	Almond & Vanilla Keto Cheesecake (Page No. 53)	Fried Chicken Recipe (Page No. 74)
Saturday	Keto Coffee Recipe (Page No. 25)	Green Keto Smoothie (Page No. 50)	Keto pizza chaffles (Page No. 88)

35-Days Keto Diet Weight Loss Challenge

Fifth Week Meal Plan

Day	Breakfast	Lunch	Dinner
Sunday	Keto Coffee Recipe (Page No. 25)	Creamy Tuscan Garlic Chicken (Page No. 51)	Chicken and Snap (Page No. 78)
Monday	Keto Coffee Recipe (Page No. 25)	Chewy Coconut Chunks (Page No. 52)	Keto pizza chaffles (Page No. 88)
Tuesday	Butter Coffee (Page No. 25)	Low Carb Smoothie (Page No. 50)	Chicken salad with guacamole (Page No. 80)
Wednesday	Egg Medley Muffins (Page No. 27)	Keto Avocado Smoothie (Page No. 51)	Baked Eggs and Zoodles (Page No. 74)
Thursday	Butter Coffee (Page No. 25)	Almond & Vanilla Keto Cheesecake (Page No. 53)	Keto chicken casserole (Page No. 78)
Friday	Cheese Omelette (Page No. 26)	Low Carb Smoothie (Page No. 50)	Fried Chicken Recipe (Page No. 74)
Saturday	Keto Coffee Recipe (Page No. 25)	Charming Keto Carrot Cake (Page No. 53)	Keto chicken enchilada bowl (Page No. 77)

Breakfast Recipes

Butter Coffee

Made for: Breakfast | Prep Time: 5 minutes | Servings: 01 people
Nutrition Per Servings: Kcal: 330, Protein: 0g, Fat: 37g, Net Carb: 0g

INGREDIENTS

- ❖ 1 cup hot coffee freshly brewed
- ❖ 2 tbsp unsalted butter
- ❖ 1 tbsp MCT oil or coconut oil

INSTRUCTIONS

1. Combine all ingredients in a blender. Blend until smooth and frothy.
2. Serve immediately.

Keto Coffee Recipe

Made for: Breakfast | Prep Time: 8 minutes | Servings: 01 people
Nutrition Per Servings: Kcal: 200, Protein: 0g, Fat: 22g, Net Carb: 0g

INGREDIENTS

- ❖ 12 oz freshly brewed coffee
- ❖ 1-2 tbsp Butter
- ❖ 1/4 tsp liquid stevia

INSTRUCTIONS

1. Add all ingredients to a blender jar and blend for 10 seconds.
2. Carefully remove the lid and pour into a coffee mug. See notes for other blending options.

Low Carb Keto Coffee Recipe

Made for: Breakfast | Prep Time: 5 minutes | Servings: 01 people
Nutrition Per Servings: Kcal: 190, Protein: 02g, Fat: 21g, Net Carb: 0g

INGREDIENTS

- ❖ 1 1/2 cups brewed coffee, coolled slightly
- ❖ 1 tbsp. raw hemp seed
- ❖ 1 tsp. pure vanilla extract
- ❖ 1 - 2 tbsp. MCT oil
- ❖ pure liquid stevia to taste

INSTRUCTIONS

1. Place all ingredients in a blender.
2. Blend for 1-2 minutes on high.
3. Pour into a mug and enjoy!

Coffee Egg Latte

Made for: Breakfast | Prep Time: 15 minutes | Servings: 01 people
Nutrition Per Servings: Kcal: 331, Protein: 24g, Fat: 25g, Net Carb: 1g

INGREDIENTS

- ❖ 8 ounces black coffee
- ❖ 1 tablespoon
- ❖ grass-fed butter
- ❖ 1 teaspoon Brain
- ❖ Octane Oil

- ❖ 2 pasture-raised eggs
- ❖ 1 scoop Vanilla
- ❖ Collagen Protein
- ❖ 1/4 teaspoon of
- ❖ Cinnamon

INSTRUCTIONS

1. Add eggs, butter, oil and cinnamon to the blender.
2. Add coffee and blend for 45 seconds on high.
3. Add collagen protein and blend for 5 seconds on low.
4. Top with cinnamon.

Cheese Omelette

Made for: Breakfast | Prep Time: 15 minutes | Servings: 01 people
Nutrition Per Servings: Kcal: 511, Protein: 24g, Fat: 43g, Net Carb: 5g

INGREDIENTS

- ❖ 3 large mushrooms (sliced).
- ❖ 3 large eggs.
- ❖ 1 oz cheddar cheese (grated).
- ❖ 1 oz butter.
- ❖ ¼ onion (finely sliced).

- ❖ Pinch salt and pepper.

INSTRUCTIONS

1. In a bowl, whisk together the eggs, salt and pepper.
2. In a large frying pan, melt the butter and fry onions and mushrooms until tender.
3. Pour in the egg mixture so that it surrounds the onions and mushrooms.
4. As the sides begin to firm and it is still slightly runny in the middle, sprinkle on the cheese.
5. Continue cooking until egg mixture is completely formed and cooked through.

Egg Medley Muffins

Made for: Breakfast | Prep Time: 15 minutes | Servings: 04 people
Nutrition Per Servings: Kcal: 335, Protein: 22g, Fat: 28g, Net Carb: 2g

INGREDIENTS

- ❖ 12 large eggs.
- ❖ 1 onion (finely chopped).
- ❖ 6 oz cheddar cheese (grated).
- ❖ 5 oz bacon (cooked and diced).
- ❖ Pinch salt and pepper.

INSTRUCTIONS

1. Preheat the oven at 175 degrees and grease a 12-hole muffin tray.
2. Equally, place onion and bacon to the bottom of each muffin tray hole.
3. In a large bowl, whisk the eggs, cheese, salt and pepper.
4. Pour the egg mixture into each hole; on top of the onions and bacon.
5. Bake for 20-25 minutes, until browned and firm to the touch.

Bacon & Cheese Egg Wrap

Made for: Breakfast | Prep Time: 25 minutes | Servings: 02 people
Nutrition Per Servings: Kcal: 413, Protein: 21g, Fat: 35g, Net Carb: 4g

INGREDIENTS

- ❖ 3 large eggs.
- ❖ 5 oz bacon (cooked and diced).

- ❖ 1 oz cheddar cheese (grated).
- ❖ 1 tbsp tomato sauce (low carb).

INSTRUCTIONS

1. In a large bowl, whisk the eggs until smooth.
2. Heat a large non-stick frying pan and slowly pour in half of the egg mixture; ensuring it reaches the edge of the pan.
3. Cook until the edges begin to brown and crisp, flip and cook the other side for an additional 30-40 seconds. Repeat with remaining egg mixture.
4. Spread the cooked egg with tomato sauce and fill with cheese and bacon; roll into an egg wrap.

Scrambled eggs with basil and butter

Made for: Breakfast | Prep Time: 15 minutes | Servings: 02 people
Nutrition Per Servings: Kcal: 625, Protein: 40g, Fat: 60g, Net Carb: 4g

INGREDIENTS

- ❖ 4 tbsp butter
- ❖ 4 eggs
- ❖ 4 tbsp heavy whipping cream
- ❖ salt and ground black pepper
- ❖ 4 oz. shredded cheese
- ❖ 4 tbsp fresh basil

INSTRUCTIONS

1. Melt butter in a pan on low heat.
2. Add cracked eggs, cream, shredded cheese, and seasoning to a small bowl. Give it a light whisk and add to the pan.
3. Stir with a spatula from the edge towards the center until the eggs are scrambled. If you prefer it soft and creamy, stir on lower heat until desired consistency.
4. Top with fresh basil.

Breakfast with Green Sauce

Made for: Breakfast | Prep Time: 25 minutes | Servings: 02 people
Nutrition Per Servings: Kcal: 384, Protein:32g, Fat: 14g, Net Carb: 3g

INGREDIENTS

- ❖ 1 cup baby spinach (baby kale)
- ❖ 1 cup arugula
- ❖ 1 cup parsley (or cilantro or basil
- ❖ etc.)
- ❖ 5 medium garlic cloves
- ❖ 5 tbsp. of hemp hearts
- ❖ 1 cup olive oil
- ❖ 5 slices bacon
- ❖ 2 eggs
- ❖ 20 asparagus tips
- ❖ Salt to taste
- ❖ pepper to taste

INSTRUCTIONS

1. Green Sauce: Combine baby spinach, arugula, parsley, garlic cloves, hemp hearts and olive oil in a blender or food processor and blend on low until well combined and almost smooth. Set aside.
2. On a sheet pan arrange your bacon slices into rings, arrange the rings in a circle.
3. Pop the sheet pan in the oven and set it to 350F. When the oven comes to temperature, remove the sheet pan from the oven (don't turn it off). Tuck 4 asparagus tips into each bacon ring.
4. Move your bacon rings closer together if needed, and then crack two eggs in between them.
5. Add your green sauce, sprinkle a little salt and pepper and pop back in the oven for 20 minutes.
6. Remove from the oven, and dig in! No need for plates. Makes enough for two!

Crustless Quiche Recipe

Made for: Breakfast | Prep Time: 35 minutes | Servings: 06 people
Nutrition Per Servings: Kcal: 216, Protein:12g, Fat: 17g, Net Carb: 4g

INGREDIENTS

- ❖ 1/2 cup bacon chopped
- ❖ 1/2 cup broccoli chopped
- ❖ 1/2 cup cherry tomatoes chopped
- ❖ 1/2 cup milk
- ❖ 1/2 cup half and half
- ❖ 2/3 cup shredded mozzarella cheese
- ❖ 5 eggs
- ❖ 1/2 tsp salt adjust to taste
- ❖ 1/4 tsp ground black pepper adjust to taste

INSTRUCTIONS

1. Preheat the oven to 325F.
2. Spray a 9-inch baking dish with cooking spray. Spread broccoli, tomatoes and bacon pieces evenly on the baking dish.
3. In a separate bowl, combine together eggs, milk, half-and-half, salt and pepper. Whisk until you get a smooth, even mixture.
4. Pour egg mixture over the veggies. Sprinkle with cheese.
5. Bake for about 25 minutes, or until the quiche is fully cooked through.
6. Let the quiche rest for a few minutes before serving. Enjoy!

Green eggs

Made for: Breakfast | Prep Time: 25 minutes | Servings: 02 people
Nutrition Per Servings: Kcal: 300, Protein:18g, Fat: 20g, Net Carb: 7g

INGREDIENTS

- ❖ 1½ tbsp rapeseed oil , plus a splash extra
- ❖ 2 trimmed leeks , sliced
- ❖ 2 garlic cloves , sliced
- ❖ ½ tsp coriander seeds
- ❖ ½ tsp fennel seeds

- ❖ pinch of chilli flakes , plus extra to serve
- ❖ 200g spinach
- ❖ 2 large eggs
- ❖ 2 tbsp Greek yogurt
- ❖ squeeze of lemo

INSTRUCTIONS

1. Heat the oil in a large frying pan. Add the leeks and a pinch of salt, then cook until soft. Add the garlic, coriander, fennel and chilli flakes. Once the seeds begin to crackle, tip in the spinach and turn down the heat. Stir everything together until the spinach has wilted and reduced, then scrape it over to one side of the pan. Pour a little oil into the pan, then crack in the eggs and fry until cooked to your liking.
2. Stir the yogurt through the spinach mix and season. Pile onto two plates, top with the fried egg, squeeze over a little lemon and season with black pepper and chilli flakes to serve.

Mexican egg roll

Made for: Breakfast | Prep Time: 15 minutes | Servings: 02 people
Nutrition Per Servings: Kcal: 132, Protein:10g, Fat: 9g, Net Carb: 1g

INGREDIENTS

- ❖ 1 large egg

- ❖ a little rapeseed oil for frying
- ❖ 2 tbsp tomato salsa
- ❖ about 1 tbsp fresh coriander

INSTRUCTIONS

1. Beat the egg with 1 tbsp water. Heat the oil in a medium non-stick pan. Add the egg and swirl round the base of the pan, as though you are making a pancake, and cook until set. There is no need to turn it.
1. Carefully tip the pancake onto a board, spread with the salsa, sprinkle with the coriander, then roll it up. It can be eaten warm or cold – you can keep it for 2 days in the fridge.

Masala frittata with avocado salsa

Made for: Breakfast | Prep Time: 40 minutes | Servings: 02 people
Nutrition Per Servings: Kcal: 350, Protein:16g, Fat: 20g, Net Carb: 7g

INGREDIENTS

- ❖ 2 tbsp rapeseed oil
- ❖ 3 onions, 2½ thinly sliced, ½ finely chopped
- ❖ 1 tbsp Madras curry paste
- ❖ 500g cherry tomatoes, halved
- ❖ 1 red chilli, deseeded and finely chopped
- ❖ small pack coriander, roughly chopped
- ❖ 8 large eggs, beaten
- ❖ 1 avocado, stoned, peeled and cubed
- ❖ juice 1 lemon

INSTRUCTIONS

1. Heat the oil in a medium non-stick, ovenproof frying pan. Tip in the sliced onions and cook over a medium heat for about 10 mins until soft and golden. Add the Madras paste and fry for 1 min more, then tip in half the tomatoes and half the chilli. Cook until the mixture is thick and the tomatoes have all burst.
3. Heat the grill to high. Add half the coriander to the eggs and season, then pour over the spicy onion mixture. Stir gently once or twice, then cook over a low heat for 8-10 mins until almost set. Transfer to the grill for 3-5 mins until set.
4. To make the salsa, mix the avocado, remaining chilli and tomatoes, chopped onion, remaining coriander and the lemon juice together, then season and serve with the frittata.

Baked Eggs

Made for: Breakfast | Prep Time: 25 minutes | Servings: 02 people
Nutrition Per Servings: Kcal: 338, Protein: 21g, Fat: 24g, Net Carb: 5g

INGREDIENTS

- ❖ 4 Eggs
- ❖ 4 Slices Bacon
- ❖ Salt and Pepper to taste 1 Oz Cheddar
- ❖ 1 Small Onion (80g)

INSTRUCTIONS

1. Fry four slices of bacon
2. Cut a small onion in half and fry
3. In a ramekin or equivalent oven-proof bowl, place onion and bacon
4. Crack two eggs into each container, making sure to not break yolk
5. Add salt and pepper
6. Add cheddar cheese
7. Bake at 350 degrees for 20 minutes or until eggs have set

Bacon & avocado frittata

Made for: Breakfast | Prep Time: 35 minutes | Servings: 04 people
Nutrition Per Servings: Kcal: 470, Protein:22g, Fat: 40g, Net Carb: 6g

INGREDIENTS

- ❖ 8 rashers smoked streaky bacon
- ❖ 3 tbsp olive oil
- ❖ 6 eggs , beaten
- ❖ 1 large avocado , halved, stoned, peeled and cut into chunky slices
- ❖ 1 small red chilli , finely chopped
- ❖ 1 heaped tsp Dijon mustard
- ❖ 2 tsp red wine vinegar
- ❖ 200g bag mixed salad leaves (we used watercress, rocket & spinach)
- ❖ 12 baby plum tomatoes , halved

INSTRUCTIONS

1. Heat a 24cm non-stick ovenproof pan and fry the bacon rashers in batches on a high heat until cooked through and crisp. Chop 4 roughly and break the other 4 into large pieces. Set aside on kitchen paper and clean the pan.

5. Heat the grill to high. Warm 1 tbsp oil in the pan. Season the eggs, add the chopped bacon and pour into the pan. Cook on a low heat for around 8 mins or until almost set. Arrange the avocado slices and bacon shards on top. Grill briefly for about 4 mins until set.

6. Mix the remaining oil, the chilli, mustard, vinegar and seasoning in a large bowl. Toss in the salad leaves and tomatoes. Serve alongside the frittata, cut into wedges.

Tomato baked eggs

Made for: Breakfast | Prep Time: 60 minutes | Servings: 04 people
Nutrition Per Servings: Kcal: 204, Protein: 09g, Fat: 16g, Net Carb: 4g

INGREDIENTS

- ❖ 900g ripe vine tomatoes
- ❖ 3 garlic cloves
- ❖ 3 tbsp olive oil
- ❖ 4 large free range eggs
- ❖ 2 tbsp chopped parsley and/or chives

INSTRUCTIONS

1. Preheat the oven to fan 180C/ conventional 200C/gas 6. Cut the tomatoes into quarters or thick wedges, depending on their size, then spread them over a fairly shallow 1.5 litre ovenproof dish. Peel the garlic, slice thinly and sprinkle over the tomatoes. Drizzle with the olive oil, season well with salt and pepper and stir everything together until the tomatoes are glistening.

2. Slide the dish into the oven and bake for 40 minutes until the tomatoes have softened and are tinged with brown.

3. Make four gaps among the tomatoes, break an egg into each gap and cover the dish with a sheet of foil. Return it to the oven for 5-10 minutes until the eggs are set to your liking. Scatter over the herbs and serve piping hot with thick slices of toast or warm ciabatta and a green salad on the side.

Mushroom baked eggs with squished tomatoes

Made for: Breakfast | Prep Time: 35 minutes | Servings: 02 people
Nutrition Per Servings: Kcal: 147, Protein: 12g, Fat: 08g, Net Carb: 05g

INGREDIENTS

- ❖ 2 large flat mushrooms (about 85g each), stalks removed and chopped
- ❖ rapeseed oil , for brushing
- ❖ ½ garlic clove , grated (optional)

- ❖ a few thyme leaves
- ❖ 2 tomatoes , halved
- ❖ 2 large eggs
- • 2 handfuls rocket

INSTRUCTIONS

1. Heat oven to 200C/180C fan/gas 6. Brush the mushrooms with a little oil and the garlic (if using). Place the mushrooms in two very lightly greased gratin dishes, bottom-side up, and season lightly with pepper. Top with the chopped stalks and thyme, cover with foil and bake for 20 mins.

2. Remove the foil, add the tomatoes to the dishes and break an egg carefully onto each of the mushrooms. Season and add a little more thyme, if you like. Return to the oven for 10-12 mins or until the eggs are set but the yolks are still runny. Top with the rocket and eat straight from the dishes.

One-pan egg & veg brunch

Made for: Breakfast | Prep Time: 30 minutes | Servings: 04 people
Nutrition Per Servings: Kcal: 170, Protein: 09g, Fat: 07g, Net Carb: 10g

INGREDIENTS

- ❖ 300g baby new potatoes , halved
- ❖ ½ tbsp rapeseed oil
- ❖ 1 knob of butter
- ❖ 1 courgette , cut into small chunks
- ❖ 1 yellow pepper , cut into small chunks
- ❖ 1 red pepper , cut into small chunks

- ❖ 2 spring onions , finely sliced
- ❖ 1 garlic clove , crushed
- ❖ 1 sprig thyme , leaves picked
- ❖ 4 eggs
- ❖ toast , to serv

INSTRUCTIONS

1. Boil the new potatoes for 8 mins, then drain.

2. Heat the oil and butter in a large non-stick frying pan, then add the courgette, peppers, potatoes and a little salt and pepper. Cook for 10 mins, stirring from time to time until everything is starting to brown. Add the spring onions, garlic and thyme and cook for 2 mins more.

3. Make four spaces in the pan and crack in the eggs. Cover with foil or a lid and cook for around 4 mins, or until the eggs are cooked (with the yolks soft for dipping into). Sprinkle with more thyme leaves and ground black pepper if you like. Serve with toast.

Baked eggs brunch

Made for: Breakfast | Prep Time: 40 minutes | Servings: 04 people
Nutrition Per Servings: Kcal: 210, Protein: 12g, Fat: 13g, Net Carb: 10g

INGREDIENTS

- 2 tbsp olive oil
- 2 leeks , thinly sliced
- 2 onions , thinly sliced
- 2 x 100g bags baby spinach leaves
- handful fresh wholemeal breadcrumbs

- 25g parmesan (or vegetarian alternative), finely grated
- 4 sundried tomatoes , chopped
- 4 medium eggs

INSTRUCTIONS

1. Heat oven to 200C/180C fan/gas 6. Heat the oil in a pan and add the leeks, onions and seasoning. Cook for 15-20 mins until soft and beginning to caramelise.
2. Meanwhile, put the spinach in a colander and pour over a kettle of boiling water. When cool enough to handle, squeeze out as much liquid as possible. Mix the breadcrumbs and cheese together.
3. Arrange the leek and onion mixture between 4 ovenproof dishes, then scatter with the spinach and pieces of sundried tomato. Make a well in the middle of each dish and crack an egg in it. Season and sprinkle with cheese crumbs. Put the dishes on a baking tray and cook for 12-15 mins, until the whites are set and yolks are cooked to your liking.

Veggie breakfast bakes

Made for: Breakfast | Prep Time: 45 minutes | Servings: 04 people
Nutrition Per Servings: Kcal: 127, Protein: 09g, Fat: 08g, Net Carb: 05g

INGREDIENTS

- 4 large field mushrooms
- 8 tomatoes , halved
- 1 garlic clove , thinly sliced

- 2 tsp olive oil
- 200g bag spinach
- 4 eggs

INSTRUCTIONS

1. Heat oven to 200C/180C fan/gas 6. Put the mushrooms and tomatoes into 4 ovenproof dishes. Divide garlic between the dishes, drizzle over the oil and some seasoning, then bake for 10 mins.

2. Meanwhile, put the spinach into a large colander, then pour over a kettle of boiling water to wilt it. Squeeze out any excess water, then add the spinach to the dishes. Make a little gap between the vegetables and crack an egg into each dish. Return to the oven and cook for a further 8-10 mins or until the egg is cooked to your liking.

Mushroom brunch

Made for: Breakfast | Prep Time: 20 minutes | Servings: 04 people
Nutrition Per Servings: Kcal: 154, Protein: 13g, Fat: 11g, Net Carb: 01g

INGREDIENTS

- ❖ 250g mushrooms
- ❖ 1 garlic clove
- ❖ 1 tbsp olive oil

- ❖ 160g bag kale
- ❖ 4 eggs

INSTRUCTIONS

1. Slice the mushrooms and crush the garlic clove. Heat the olive oil in a large non-stick frying pan, then fry the garlic over a low heat for 1 min. Add the mushrooms and cook until soft. Then, add the kale. If the kale won't all fit in the pan, add half and stir until wilted, then add the rest. Once all the kale is wilted, season.

2. Now crack in the eggs and keep them cooking gently for 2-3 mins. Then, cover with the lid to for a further 2-3 mins or until the eggs are cooked to your liking. Serve with bread.

Herby Persian frittata

Made for: Breakfast | Prep Time: 20 minutes | Servings: 02 people
Nutrition Per Servings: Kcal: 198, Protein: 14g, Fat: 11g, Net Carb: 09g

INGREDIENTS

- ❖ 3 eggs
- ❖ ½ tsp baking powder
- ❖ ¼ tsp turmeric
- ❖ 1 small pack of coriander and parsley, roughly chopped
- ❖ ½ small pack dill , roughly chopped
- ❖ 4 spring onions , thinly sliced

- ❖ 1 tbsp currants or barberries, if you can find them
- ❖ 1 tbsp toasted walnuts (optional), roughly chopped
- ❖ 1 tbsp cold pressed rapeseed oil
- ❖ 30g feta , crumbled

INSTRUCTIONS

1. Heat grill to high. Whisk the eggs together in a large bowl, add the baking powder and turmeric, then season with salt and pepper. Stir in most of the herbs, then add the spring onions, currants and walnuts.

2. Drizzle the oil into a small ovenproof, non-stick frying pan over a medium heat. Pour in the herby egg mixture and cook for 8-10 mins until the egg is nearly set, then put the frittata under the grill for a final minute until cooked through. Sprinkle over the remaining herbs and the crumbled feta to serve.

Crustless Quiche Recipe

Made for: Breakfast | Prep Time: 35 minutes | Servings: 04 people

Nutrition Per Servings: Kcal: 337, Protein: 22g, Fat: 20g, Net Carb: 12g

INGREDIENTS

- ❖ 3 tbsp olive oil
- ❖ 2 leeks , washed and sliced
- ❖ 200g bag baby spinach
- ❖ 250g frozen peas
- ❖ 2 fat garlic cloves , finely chopped
- ❖ 1 tbsp cumin seeds
- ❖ small pack parsley , roughly chopped
- ❖ small pack coriander , roughly chopped

- ❖ small pack mint , leaves picked and roughly chopped, reserving a few leaves to garnish
- ❖ 8 medium eggs
- ❖ 150g pot natural yogurt
- ❖ 1 tbsp harissa
- ❖ flatbread , to serve

INSTRUCTIONS

1. Heat the oil in a wide, shallow frying pan over a medium heat. Add the leeks with a pinch of salt and cook for 4 mins until softened. Add handfuls of spinach to the pan, stirring until wilted.

2. Stir in the peas, garlic, cumin, herbs and some seasoning. Cook for a few mins until it smells fragrant, then create four gaps and crack two eggs into each. Cover and cook for 10 mins or until the whites are set but the yolks are runny – they will carry on cooking slightly as you take them to the table.

3. Season the eggs with flaky sea salt, dollop spoonfuls of the yogurt interspersed with the harissa, and scatter over a few mint leaves. Serve with a pile of flatbread for scooping.

Eggs with basil, spinach & tomatoes

Made for: Breakfast | Prep Time: 10 minutes | Servings: 02 people
Nutrition Per Servings: Kcal: 298, Protein: 20g, Fat: 19g, Net Carb: 10g

INGREDIENTS

- ❖ 1 tbsp rapeseed oil , plus 1 tsp
- ❖ 3 tomatoes , halved
- ❖ 4 large eggs
- ❖ 4 tbsp natural bio yogurt

- ❖ ⅓ small pack basil , chopped
- ❖ 175g baby spinach , dried well (if it needs washing)

INSTRUCTIONS

1. Heat 1 tsp oil in a large non-stick frying pan, add the tomatoes and cook, cut-side down, over a medium heat. While they are cooking, beat the eggs in a jug with the yogurt, 2 tbsp water, plenty of black pepper and the basil.

2. Transfer the tomatoes to serving plates. Add the spinach to the pan and wilt, stirring a few times while you cook the eggs.

3. Heat the rest of the oil in a non-stick pan over a medium heat, pour in the egg mixture and stir every now and then until scrambled and just set. Spoon the spinach onto the plates and top with the scrambled eggs.

Herb omelette with fried tomatoes

Made for: Breakfast | Prep Time: 10 minutes | Servings: 02 people
Nutrition Per Servings: Kcal: 204, Protein: 17g, Fat: 13g, Net Carb: 04g

INGREDIENTS

- ❖ 1 tsp rapeseed oil
- ❖ 3 tomatoes , halved
- ❖ 4 large eggs

- ❖ 1 tbsp chopped parsley
- ❖ 1 tbsp chopped basil

INSTRUCTIONS

1. Heat the oil in a small non-stick frying pan, then cook the tomatoes cut-side down until starting to soften and colour. Meanwhile, beat the eggs with the herbs and plenty of freshly ground black pepper in a small bowl.

2. Scoop the tomatoes from the pan and put them on two serving plates. Pour the egg mixture into the pan and stir gently with a wooden spoon so the egg that sets on the base of the pan moves to enable uncooked egg to flow into the space. Stop stirring when it's nearly cooked to allow it to set into an omelette. Cut into four and serve with the tomatoes.

Skinny pepper, tomato & ham omelette

Made for: Breakfast | Prep Time: 25 minutes | Servings: 02 people
Nutrition Per Servings: Kcal: 204, Protein: 21g, Fat: 12g, Net Carb: 05g

INGREDIENTS

- ❖ 2 whole eggs and 3 egg whites
- ❖ 1 tsp olive oil
- ❖ 1 red pepper , deseeded and finely chopped
- ❖ 2 spring onions , white and green parts kept separate and finely chopped
- ❖ few slices wafer-thin extra-lean ham , shredded
- ❖ 25g reduced-fat mature cheddar
- ❖ wholemeal toast , to serve (optional)
- ❖ 1-2 chopped fresh tomatoes , to serve (optional)

INSTRUCTIONS

1. Mix the eggs and egg whites with some seasoning and set aside. Heat the oil in a medium non-stick frying pan and cook the pepper for 3-4 mins. Throw in the white parts of the spring onions and cook for 1 min more. Pour in the eggs and cook over a medium heat until almost completely set.
2. Sprinkle on the ham and cheese and continue cooking until just set in the centre, or flash it under a hot grill if you like it more well done. Serve straight from the pan with the green part of the spring onion sprinkled on top, the chopped tomato and some wholemeal toast.

Mushroom & basil omelette with smashed tomato

Made for: Breakfast | Prep Time: 20 minutes | Servings: 02 people
Nutrition Per Servings: Kcal: 196, Protein: 14g, Fat: 14g, Net Carb: 04g

INGREDIENTS

- ❖ 2 tomatoes , halved
- ❖ 3 medium eggs
- ❖ 1 tbsp snipped chive
- ❖ 300g chestnut mushroom , sliced
- ❖ 1 tsp unsalted butter
- ❖ 2 tbsp low-fat cream cheese
- ❖ 1 tbsp finely chopped basil leaves

INSTRUCTIONS

1. Heat the grill to its highest setting and place the tomatoes on a square of foil underneath, turning occasionally to prevent burning. When the tomatoes are slightly scorched, remove from the grill, squashing them slightly to release the juices.

2. Break the eggs into a bowl and mix with a fork. Add a small splash of water and mix. Add the chives and some black pepper, and beat some more. Set aside while you prepare the mushrooms.

3. In a non-stick frying pan, heat the butter over a medium heat until foaming. Add the mushrooms and cook for 5-8 mins until tender, stirring every few mins. Remove and set aside.

4. Briskly stir the egg mixture, then add to the hot pan (tilting it so that the mixture covers the entire base) and leave for 10 secs or so until it begins to set. With a fork, gently stir the egg here and there so that any unset mixture gets cooked.

5. While the egg mixture is still slightly loose, spoon the mushroom mix onto one side of the omelette, and top with the cream cheese and basil leaves. Flip the other side of the omelette over to cover, if you like. Leave to cook for 1 min more, then cut in half and slide each half onto a plate. Serve immediately with the tomatoes on the side.

Egg with bacon & asparagus soldiers

Made for: Breakfast | Prep Time: 35 minutes | Servings: 04 people
Nutrition Per Servings: Kcal: 306, Protein: 20g, Fat: 19g, Net Carb: 14g

INGREDIENTS

- ❖ 8 asparagus spears (about 300g), woody ends discarded
- ❖ 4 long thin slices rustic bread (preferably sourdough)
- ❖ 8 rashers smoked streaky bacon or pancetta
- ❖ 4 duck eggs

INSTRUCTIONS

1. Heat your grill to high. Snap off the woody ends of the asparagus spears and discard. Cut the bread into 12 soldiers, a little shorter than the asparagus.

2. Place a spear onto each soldier and wrap tightly with a rasher of bacon. Place on a baking tray, season and grill for 15 mins or until the bacon is crisp.

3. Bring a pan of salted water to the boil and simmer the duck eggs for about 7 mins, to get a runny yolk and a cooked white. Serve immediately with the warm soldiers for dipping.

Eggs with pancetta avocado soldiers

Made for: Breakfast | Prep Time: 15 minutes | Servings: 02 people
Nutrition Per Servings: Kcal: 517, Protein: 22g, Fat: 46g, Net Carb: 01g

INGREDIENTS

- ❖ 4 eggs
- ❖ 1 tbsp vegetable oil
- ❖ 1 ripe avocado , cut into slices
- ❖ 100g smoked pancetta rashers

INSTRUCTIONS

1. Bring a large saucepan of salted water to the boil. Carefully drop the eggs into the water and boil for 5 mins for runny yolks.
2. Meanwhile, heat the oil in a non-stick pan and wrap each avocado slice in pancetta. Fry for 2-3 mins over a high heat until cooked and crisp.
3. Serve the eggs in egg cups with the pancetta avocado soldiers on the side for dipping.

Mushroom hash with poached eggs

Made for: Breakfast | Prep Time: 30 minutes | Servings: 04 people
Nutrition Per Servings: Kcal: 283, Protein: 15g, Fat: 17g, Net Carb: 12g

INGREDIENTS

- ❖ 1 ½ tbsp rapeseed oil
- ❖ 2 large onions , halved and sliced
- ❖ 500g closed cup mushrooms , quartered
- ❖ 1 tbsp fresh thyme leaves , plus extra for sprinkling
- ❖ 500g fresh tomatoes , chopped
- ❖ 1 tsp smoked paprika
- ❖ 4 tsp omega seed mix (see tip)
- ❖ 4 large eggs

INSTRUCTIONS

1. Heat the oil in a large non-stick frying pan and fry the onions for a few mins. Cover the pan and leave the onions to cook in their own steam for 5 mins more.
2. Tip in the mushrooms with the thyme and cook, stirring frequently, for 5 mins until softened. Add the tomatoes and paprika, cover the pan and cook for 5 mins until pulpy. Stir through the seed mix.

3. If you're making this recipe as part of our two-person Summer Healthy Diet Plan, poach two of the eggs in lightly simmering water to your liking. Serve on top of half the hash with a sprinkling of fresh thyme and some black pepper. Chill the remaining hash to warm in a pan and eat with freshly poached eggs on another day. If you're serving four people, poach all four eggs, divide the hash between four plates, sprinkle with thyme and black pepper and serve with the eggs on top.

Breakfast burrito

Made for: Breakfast | Prep Time: 25 minutes | Servings: 01 people
Nutrition Per Servings: Kcal: 361, Protein: 16g, Fat: 21g, Net Carb: 26g

INGREDIENTS

- ❖ 1 tsp chipotle paste
- ❖ 1 egg
- ❖ 1 tsp rapeseed oil
- ❖ 50g kale
- ❖ 7 cherry tomatoes, halved
- ❖ ½ small avocado, sliced
- ❖ 1 wholemeal tortilla wrap, warmed

INSTRUCTIONS

1. Whisk the chipotle paste with the egg and some seasoning in a jug. Heat the oil in a large frying pan, add the kale and tomatoes.
2. Cook until the kale is wilted and the tomatoes have softened, then push everything to the side of the pan. Pour the beaten egg into the cleared half of the pan and scramble. Layer everything into the centre of your wrap, topping with the avocado, then wrap up and eat immediately.

Breakfast egg wraps

Made for: Breakfast | Prep Time: 15 minutes | Servings: 04 people
Nutrition Per Servings: Kcal: 429, Protein: 28g, Fat: 20g, Net Carb: 31g

INGREDIENTS

- ❖ 500g pack closed cup mushrooms
- ❖ 4 tsp cold pressed rapeseed oil , plus 2 drops
- ❖ 320g cherry tomatoes , halved, or 8 tomatoes, cut into wedges
- ❖ 2 generous handfuls parsley , finely chopped
- ❖ 8 tbsp porridge oats (40g)
- ❖ 10 eggs
- ❖ 4 tsp English mustard powder made up with water

INSTRUCTIONS

1. Thickly slice half the pack of mushrooms. Heat 2 tsp rapeseed oil in a non-stick pan. Add the mushrooms, stir briefly then fry with the lid on the pan for 6-8 mins. Stir in half the tomatoes then cook 1-2 mins more with the lid off until softened.

2. Beat together the eggs really well with the parsley and oats. Heat a drop of oil in a large non-stick frying pan. Pour in a ¼ of the egg mix and fry for 1 min until almost set, flip over as if making a pancake. Tip from the pan, spread with a quarter of the mustard, spoon a ¼ the filling down the centre and roll up. Now make a second wrap using another ¼ of the egg mix and filling. If you're following our Healthy Diet Plan, save the rest for the following day.

Green shakshuka

Made for: Breakfast | Prep Time: 35 minutes | Servings: 04 people
Nutrition Per Servings: Kcal: 337, Protein: 22g, Fat: 20g, Net Carb: 10g

INGREDIENTS

- 3 tbsp olive oil
- 2 leeks , washed and sliced
- 200g bag baby spinach
- 250g frozen peas
- 2 fat garlic cloves , finely chopped
- 1 tbsp cumin seeds
- small pack parsley , roughly chopped
- small pack coriander , roughly chopped

- small pack mint , leaves picked and roughly chopped, reserving a few leaves to garnish
- 8 medium eggs
- 150g pot natural yogurt
- 1 tbsp harissa
- flatbread , to serve

INSTRUCTIONS

1. Heat the oil in a wide, shallow frying pan over a medium heat. Add the leeks with a pinch of salt and cook for 4 mins until softened. Add handfuls of spinach to the pan, stirring until wilted.

2. Stir in the peas, garlic, cumin, herbs and some seasoning. Cook for a few mins until it smells fragrant, then create four gaps and crack two eggs into each. Cover and cook for 10 mins or until the whites are set but the yolks are runny – they will carry on cooking slightly as you take them to the table.

3. Season the eggs with flaky sea salt, dollop spoonfuls of the yogurt interspersed with the harissa, and scatter over a few mint leaves. Serve with a pile of flatbread for scooping.

Sprout & spinach baked eggs

Made for: Breakfast | Prep Time: 20 minutes | Servings: 04 people
Nutrition Per Servings: Kcal: 268, Protein: 21g, Fat: 15g, Net Carb: 10g

INGREDIENTS

- ❖ 1 tbsp olive oil
- ❖ 1 tsp cumin seeds
- ❖ 1 onion , chopped
- ❖ 2 garlic cloves , crushed
- ❖ 1 green chilli , chopped (deseeded if you don't want it very hot)
- ❖ 300g Brussels sprouts , roughly shredded
- ❖ 450g spinach
- ❖ ½ lemon , juiced
- ❖ 6 eggs
- ❖ ½ small pack coriander , yogurt, sriracha and thick slices of sourdough, to serve

INSTRUCTIONS

1. Heat the oil in a frying pan with high sides, scatter in the cumin seeds and toast a little, then add the onion and fry until softened, around 5 mins. Add the garlic and chilli and fry for 1 min. Tip the sprouts into the pan and cook for 5 mins until softened, then add the spinach – you may have to do this in batches. Cook until the spinach has wilted down, then squeeze in the lemon juice to taste. Season well.

2. Use a spoon to create six holes in the greens to crack the eggs into. Break the eggs into the holes, cover the pan with a lid and cook for 5-7 mins until the eggs have set, but the yolk remains runny. Sprinkle over the coriander and serve immediately, drizzled with natural yogurt and sriracha, and with sourdough on the side.

Breakfast smoothie

Made for: Breakfast | Prep Time: 02 minutes | Servings: 02 people
Nutrition Per Servings: Kcal: 156, Protein: 04g, Fat: 03g, Net Carb: 21g

INGREDIENTS

- ❖ 1 banana
- ❖ 1 tbsp porridge oats

- ❖ 80g soft fruit (whatever you have – strawberries, blueberries, and mango all work well)
- ❖ 150ml milk
- ❖ 1 tsp honey
- ❖ 1 tsp vanilla extract

INSTRUCTIONS

1. Put all the ingredients in a blender and whizz for 1 min until smooth.
2. Pour the banana oat smoothie into two glasses to serve.

Breakfast naans

Made for: Breakfast | Prep Time: 10 minutes | Servings: 02 people
Nutrition Per Servings: Kcal: 503, Protein: 20g, Fat: 30g, Net Carb: 35g

INGREDIENTS

- ❖ 1 tbsp vegetable or sunflower oil
- ❖ 2 eggs
- ❖ 2 small naan breads
- ❖ 4 tbsp low-fat cream cheese
- ❖ 2 tbsp mango chutney
- ❖ 1 avocado , halved and sliced
- ❖ ½ lime , juiced
- ❖ 1 green chilli
- ❖ small handful coriander , leaves picked

INSTRUCTIONS

1. Heat oven to 200C/180C fan/gas 6. Heat the oil in a pan, then fry the eggs. Warm the naan breads in the oven while the eggs are cooking.
2. Spread the warm naans with the cream cheese, then drizzle with the chutney. Add a fried egg to each naan and top with the avocado, lime juice, chilli and coriander. Season and tuck in.

Chorizo & halloumi breakfast baguette

Made for: Breakfast | Prep Time: 55 minutes | Servings: 04 people
Nutrition Per Servings: Kcal: 872, Protein: 36g, Fat: 40g, Net Carb: 91g

INGREDIENTS

- 1 large avocado
- 1 lime , juiced
- 1 red onion , halved and thinly sliced
- drizzle of oil
- 150g chorizo , sliced on an angle
- 250g block halloumi , sliced into 8 pieces
- 1 large baguette or 2 smaller ones
- small bunch coriander , leaves picked

- For the tomato jam
- 400g can chopped tomatoes
- red chilli , finely chopped (deseeded if you don't want much spice)
- thumb-sized piece ginger , grated
- 1 star anise
- 250g caster sugar
- 150ml red wine vinegar

INSTRUCTIONS

1. To make the tomato jam, put all the ingredients in a pan, season and simmer for 30 mins until you have a rich, thick glossy jam. Cool, then transfer to a sterilised jar (if you want to keep for over two weeks). Will keep, unopened, for six months.
2. Halve the avocado and scoop into a bowl. Add half the lime juice and some salt and mash with a fork. Put the onion in a small bowl, pour over the rest of the lime juice and season with a pinch of salt. Mix well and set aside to lightly pickle.
3. Heat a drizzle of oil in a large frying pan. Cook the chorizo slices on one side of the pan and the halloumi on the other, turning once the halloumi is golden and the chorizo is sizzling. Cook for about 4-5 mins in total.
4. Meanwhile, split and warm the baguette in the oven. Spread the avocado over one side of the baguette, and the tomato jam over the other. Fill with the halloumi, chorizo, coriander and pickled red onions. Cut up and tuck in.

Gordon's eggs Benedict

Made for: Breakfast | Prep Time: 20 minutes | Servings: 04 people
Nutrition Per Servings: Kcal: 705, Protein: 18g, Fat: 64g, Net Carb: 16g

INGREDIENTS

- 3 tbsp white wine vinegar

- ❖ 4 large free range eggs
- ❖ 2 toasting muffins
- ❖ 1 batch hot hollandaise sauce (see 'Goes well with' below)
- ❖ 4 slices Parma ham (or Serrano or Bayonne)

INSTRUCTIONS

1. Bring a deep saucepan of water to the boil (at least 2 litres) and add 3 tbsp white wine vinegar. Break the eggs into 4 separate coffee cups or ramekins. Split the muffins, toast them and warm some plates.
2. Swirl the vinegared water briskly to form a vortex and slide in an egg. It will curl round and set to a neat round shape. Cook for 2-3 mins, then remove with a slotted spoon.
3. Repeat with the other eggs, one at a time, re-swirling the water as you slide in the eggs. Spread some sauce on each muffin, scrunch a slice of ham on top, then top with an egg. Spoon over the remaining hollandaise and serve at once.

Breakfast muffins

Made for: Breakfast | Prep Time: 45 minutes | Servings: 12 people
Nutrition Per Servings: Kcal: 179, Protein: 05g, Fat: 07g, Net Carb: 09g

INGREDIENTS

- ❖ 2 large eggs
- ❖ 150ml pot natural low-fat yogurt
- ❖ 50ml rapeseed oil
- ❖ 100g apple sauce or pureed apples (find with the baby food)
- ❖ 1 ripe banana, mashed
- ❖ 4 tbsp clear honey
- ❖ 1 tsp vanilla extract

- ❖ 200g wholemeal flour
- ❖ 50g rolled oats, plus extra for sprinkling
- ❖ 1½ tsp baking powder
- ❖ 1½ tsp bicarbonate of soda
- ❖ 1½ tsp cinnamon
- ❖ 100g blueberry
- ❖ 2 tbsp mixed seed (we used pumpkin, sunflower and flaxseed)

INSTRUCTIONS

1. Heat oven to 180C/160C fan/gas 4. Line a 12-hole muffin tin with 12 large muffin cases. In a jug, mix the eggs, yogurt, oil, apple sauce, banana, honey and vanilla. Tip the remaining ingredients, except the seeds, into a large bowl, add a pinch of salt and mix to combine.
2. Pour the wet ingredients into the dry and mix briefly until you have a smooth batter – don't overmix as this will make the muffins heavy. Divide the batter between the cases. Sprinkle the muffins with

the extra oats and the seeds. Bake for 25-30 mins until golden and well risen, and a skewer inserted into the centre of a muffin comes out clean. Remove from the oven, transfer to a wire rack and leave to cool. Can be stored in a sealed container for up to 3 days.

Keto Mexican scrambled eggs

Made for: Breakfast | Prep Time: 25 minutes | Servings: 02 people
Nutrition Per Servings: Kcal: 230, Protein: 16g, Fat: 21g, Net Carb: 2g

INGREDIENTS

- ½ oz. butter
- ½ scallion, finely chopped
- 1 pickled jalapeno, finely chopped
- ½ tomato, finely chopped
- 3 eggs
- 1½ oz. shredded cheese
- salt and pepper

INSTRUCTIONS

1. In a large frying pan, melt the butter over medium high heat.
2. Add scallions, jalapeños and tomatoes, and fry for 3-4 minutes.
3. Beat the eggs and pour into the pan. Scramble for 2 minutes. Add cheese and seasonings

Keto mushroom omelet

Made for: Breakfast | Prep Time: 20 minutes | Servings: 02 people
Nutrition Per Servings: Kcal: 230, Protein: 16g, Fat: 21g, Net Carb: 2g

INGREDIENTS

- 6 eggs
- 2 oz. butter, for frying
- 2 oz. shredded cheese
- ½ yellow onion, chopped
- 8 large mushrooms, sliced
- salt and pepper

INSTRUCTIONS

1. Crack the eggs into a mixing bowl with a pinch of salt and pepper. Whisk the eggs with a fork until smooth and frothy.
1. Melt the butter in a frying pan, over medium heat. Add the mushrooms and onion to the pan, stirring until tender, and then pour in the egg mixture, surrounding the veggies.

2. When the omelet begins to cook and get firm, but still has a little raw egg on top, sprinkle cheese over the egg.
3. Using a spatula, carefully ease around the edges of the omelet, and then fold it over in half. When it starts to turn golden brown underneath, remove the pan from the heat and slide the omelet on to a plate.

Keto deviled eggs

Made for: Breakfast | Prep Time: 15 minutes | Servings: 02 people
Nutrition Per Servings: Kcal: 170, Protein: 08g, Fat: 16g, Net Carb: 1g

INGREDIENTS

- ❖ 2 eggs
- ❖ ½ tsp tabasco
- ❖ 2 tbsp mayonnaise
- ❖ ½ pinch herbal salt

- ❖ 4 cooked and peeled shrimp
- ❖ fresh dill

INSTRUCTIONS

1. Start by boiling the eggs by placing them in a pot and covering them with water. Place the pot over medium heat and bring to a light boil.
2. Boil for 8-10 minutes to make sure the eggs are hardboiled.
3. Remove the eggs from the pot and place in an ice bath for a few minutes before peeling.
4. Split the eggs in half and scoop out the yolks.
5. Place the egg whites on a plate.
6. Mash the yolks with a fork and add tabasco, herbal salt and homemade mayonnaise.
7. Add the mixture, using two spoons, to the egg whites and top with a shrimp on each, or a piece of smoked salmon.
8. Decorate with dill.

Lunch Recipes

Green Keto Smoothie

Made for: Lunch | Prep Time: 10 minutes | Servings: 02 people
Nutrition Per Servings: Kcal: 141, Protein: 04g, Fat: 10.5g, Net Carb: 4g

INGREDIENTS

- ❖ 1 oz. kale leaves
- ❖ 1/2 avocado (peeled and stone removed)
- ❖ 1 stick celery (chopped)
- ❖ 2 oz. cucumber (peeled)
- ❖ 1 cup unsweetened almond milk (or regular milk)
- ❖ 1 tbsp. peanut butter (you can use any nut butter you like)
- ❖ 2 tbsp. freshly squeeze lemon juice

INSTRUCTIONS

1. Add all of the ingredients to a high-speed blender.
2. Pulse to combine, stopping to scrape down the sides if necessary.
3. Serve immediately garnished with fresh mint or store in the fridge for later that day.

Low Carb Smoothie

Made for: Lunch | Prep Time: 5 minutes | Servings: 01 people
Nutrition Per Servings: Kcal: 332, Protein: 10g, Fat: 32g, Net Carb: 5g

INGREDIENTS

- ❖ 1 Cup Almond Breeze Original Almondmilk
- ❖ 1 Cup Crushed ice
- ❖ 1/4 Cup Avocado (about 1/2 an avocado or 60g)
- ❖ 3 Tbsp Monkfruit, or to taste
- ❖ 2 Tbsp Natural creamy peanut butter (Almond butter for paleo)
- ❖ 1 Tbsp Unsweetened cocoa powder

INSTRUCTIONS

1. Place all ingredients into a blender and blend until smooth.
2. SLURP UP!

Keto Avocado Smoothie

Made for: Lunch | Prep Time: 5 minutes | Servings: 01 people
Nutrition Per Servings: Kcal: 316, Protein: 18g, Fat: 28g, Net Carb: 4g

INGREDIENTS

- ❖ 1/2 avocado
- ❖ 1 cup unsweetened almond milk (or milk of choice)
- ❖ 1 cup of ice
- ❖ 1 scoop keto friendly vanilla flavored protein powder

INSTRUCTIONS

1. Place all ingredients in a blender and pulse for 10-20 seconds.
2. If desired, top with additional sliced avocado, keto whipped cream, or hemp hearts.
3. Serve cold.

Creamy Tuscan Garlic Chicken

Made for: Lunch | Prep Time: 30 minutes | Servings: 03 people
Nutrition Per Servings: Kcal: 335, Protein: 19g, Fat: 26g, Net Carb: 7g

INGREDIENTS

- ❖ 1½ pounds boneless skinless chicken breasts thinly sliced
- ❖ 2 Tablespoons olive oil
- ❖ 1 cup heavy cream
- ❖ 1/2 cup chicken broth
- ❖ One teaspoon garlic powder
- ❖ One teaspoon Italian seasoning
- ❖ 1/2 cup parmesan cheese
- ❖ 1 cup spinach chopped
- ❖ 1/2 cup sun-dried tomatoes

INSTRUCTIONS

1. In a large skillet, add olive oil and cook the chicken on medium-high heat for 3-5 minutes on each side or until brown on each side and cooked until no longer pink in centre. Remove chicken and set aside on a plate.
2. Add the heavy cream, chicken broth, garlic powder, Italian seasoning, and parmesan cheese. Whisk over medium-high heat until it starts to thicken. Add the spinach and sundried tomatoes and let it simmer until the spinach begins to wilt. Add the chicken back to the pan and serve over pasta if desired.

Chewy Coconut Chunks

Made for: Lunch | Prep Time: 25 minutes | Servings: 08 people
Nutrition Per Servings: Kcal: 112, Protein: 3g, Fat: 10g, Net Carb: 6g

INGREDIENTS

- ❖ 7 oz coconut (shredded).
- ❖ ⅔ cup coconut milk (full fat).
- ❖ ¼ cup maple syrup.
- ❖ 1 tsp psyllium husk.
- ❖ ¼ tsp almond extract.
- ❖ ¼ tsp salt.

INSTRUCTIONS

1. Preheat oven at 325 degrees.
2. In a blender, mix coconut milk, maple syrup, psyllium husk, almond extract, salt, and ¾ of the coconut flakes until smooth.
3. Pour mixture into a large bowl, stir in remaining coconut flakes.
4. Line a baking tray with greaseproof paper. Using a tablespoon, scoop out chunks of the mixture and place onto the plate.
5. Bake for 30 minutes or until all chunks are golden brown.

Peanut Butter Biscuits

Made for: Lunch | Prep Time: 20 minutes | Servings: 06 people
Nutrition Per Servings: Kcal: 318, Protein: 15g, Fat: 25g, Net Carb: 7g

INGREDIENTS

- ❖ 1 cup almond flour.
- ❖ ½ cup peanut butter (unsweetened).
- ❖ ⅓ cup erythritol.
- ❖ 1 tbsp coconut oil.
- ❖ ¾ tsp baking powder.
- ❖ ½ tsp vanilla extract.

INSTRUCTIONS

1. Preheat oven at 350 degrees.
2. In a large bowl, mix all of the ingredients until a dough is formed.

3. Divide the dough into eight large biscuits.
4. Line a baking tray with greaseproof paper.
5. Bake for 10-12 minutes or until golden brown.

Charming Keto Carrot Cake

Made for: Lunch | Prep Time: 20 minutes | Servings: 02 people
Nutrition Per Servings: Kcal: 436, Protein: 17g, Fat: 38g, Net Carb: 4g

INGREDIENTS

- ¾ cup almond flour.
- ½ cup carrot (grated).
- One large egg.
- 2 tbsp cream cheese.
- 2 tbsp walnuts (finely chopped).
- 2 tbsp butter (melted).
- 2 tbsp erythritol.
- 1 tbsp thick cream.
- 2 tsp cinnamon.
- 1 tsp mixed spice.
- 1 tsp baking powder.

INSTRUCTIONS

1. In a bowl, mix almond flour, cinnamon, baking powder, erythritol, walnuts, and mixed spice.
2. Mix in the egg, butter, thick cream, and carrot until well combined.
3. Grease 2 microwave-safe ramekins and split the mixture evenly between the two.
4. Microwave on high for 5 minutes.
5. Spread cream cheese on the top.

Almond & Vanilla Keto Cheesecake

Made for: Lunch | Prep Time: 15 minutes | Servings: 03 people
Nutrition Per Servings: Kcal: 435, Protein: 10g, Fat: 44g, Net Carb: 5g

INGREDIENTS

- 16 oz cream cheese.
- 2 cups almond flour.
- One ¼ cup erythritol.
- ¾ cup of thick cream.
- ½ cup sour cream.
- ⅓ cup butter (melted).
- 2 tsp vanilla extract.

1. Mix butter, flour, ¼ cup erythritol, and 1 tsp vanilla until a dough is formed.
2. Press the dough into a 9-inch ovenproof dish and chill for 60 minutes.
3. In a blender, mix cream cheese, 1 cup erythritol, and remaining vanilla until creamy.
4. Add in the sour cream and thick cream until thickened.
5. Pour onto chilled crust and refrigerate for 4-5 hours.

Chicken Salad Stuffed Peppers

Made for: Lunch | Prep Time: 20 minutes | Servings: 02 people
Nutrition Per Servings: Kcal: 116, Protein: 13g, Fat: 18g, Net Carb: 6g

INGREDIENTS

- ⅔ cup Greek yoghurt
- Two tablespoons Dijon mustard
- Two tablespoons seasoned rice vinegar
- Kosher salt and freshly ground black Pepper
- ⅓ cup chopped fresh parsley
- Meat from 1 rotisserie chicken, cubed
- Four stalks celery, sliced
- One bunch scallions, sliced and divided
- 1-pint cherry tomatoes, quartered and divided
- ½ English cucumber, diced
- Three bell peppers halved and seeds removed

INSTRUCTIONS

1. In a medium bowl, whisk together the Greek yoghurt, mustard, and rice vinegar; season with salt and Pepper. Stir in the parsley.
2. Add the chicken, celery, and three-quarters each of the scallions, tomatoes, and cucumbers. Stir well to combine.
3. Divide the chicken salad among the bell pepper boats.
4. Garnish with the remaining scallions, tomatoes, and cucumbers.

Funky Fried Fish Cakes

Made for: Lunch | Prep Time: 30 minutes | Servings: 06 people
Nutrition Per Servings: Kcal: 198, Protein: 13g, Fat: 15g, Net Carb: 1g

INGREDIENTS

- 6 oz mackerel (smoked).
- 4 oz haddock (smoked).
- 4 oz salmon.
- One large egg.

- ❖ One garlic clove (crushed).
- ❖ 4 tbsp fresh parsley (finely chopped).
- ❖ 3 tbsp parmesan (grated).
- ❖ 1 tbsp coconut flour.
- ❖ 1 tbsp flaxseed (ground).
- ❖ 1 ½ oz butter.
- ❖ 1 tbsp coconut oil.
- ❖ 1 tsp salt.
- ❖ 1 tsp chilli flakes.

INSTRUCTIONS

1. Chop all fish into small chunks and mix.
2. In a separate bowl, mix all ingredients except olive oil, coconut oil, and butter.
3. Using your hands, squeeze the mixture until all is combined.
4. Mould the mixture into round, flat balls.
5. In a large frying pan, heat the olive oil, coconut oil, and butter.
6. Fry the fish cakes for 4-5 minutes on each side.

Gorgeous Garlic Gnocchi

Made for: Lunch | Prep Time: 20 minutes | Servings: 04 people
Nutrition Per Servings: Kcal: 334, Protein: 12g, Fat: 27g, Net Carb: 7g

INGREDIENTS

- ❖ 1 ⅓ cup almond flour.
- ❖ ⅔ cup parmesan (grated).
- ❖ ½ cup ricotta cheese.
- ❖ One large egg.
- ❖ Four garlic cloves (chopped).
- ❖ 2 tbsp coconut flour.
- ❖ 2 tbsp butter.
- ❖ 2 tbsp olive oil.
- ❖ 2 tsp xanthan gum.
- ❖ 1 tsp garlic powder.
- ❖ ¼ tsp salt.

INSTRUCTIONS

1. In a bowl, mix almond flour, coconut flour, garlic powder, and xanthan gum.
2. In a separate bowl, whisk the egg and add ricotta, parmesan, and salt; mix until well combined.
3. Add the flour mixture to the cheese mixture and mix thoroughly until the crumble becomes a sticky dough ball.
4. Wrap the dough ball in cling film and let settle in the fridge for 60 minutes.
5. Cut the dough into 1-inch pieces, moulding them into an oval shape.
6. In a large frying pan, add olive oil and butter; fry the garlic until lightly browned.
7. Fry the gnocchi for 5 minutes, spooning on the garlic oil.

Keto roast chicken with broccoli

Made for: Lunch | Prep Time: 55 minutes | Servings: 04 people
Nutrition Per Servings: Kcal: 780, Protein: 30g, Fat: 70g, Net Carb: 2g

INGREDIENTS

Chicken legs

- ❖ 4 chicken legs (about 5 oz each)
- ❖ 1 tsp garlic powder
- ❖ 2 tbsp olive oil
- ❖ 1 tbsp Italian seasoning
- ❖ ½ tsp salt (if not already salt in the Italian seasoning)

Garlic butter

- ❖ 14 tbsp unsalted butter, softened
- ❖ 2 garlic cloves, pressed
- ❖ 1 tbsp fresh parsley, finely chopped (optional)
- ❖ salt and ground black pepper, to taste
- ❖ Broccoli
- ❖ 20 oz. broccoli
- ❖ Salt

INSTRUCTIONS

1. Preheat oven to 400 °F (200 °C).
2. Toss chicken legs with olive oil and seasoning.
3. Put the chicken legs, skin side up, in a baking dish. Bake 40-45 minutes or until juices run clear and chicken reaches 165 °F (74 °C).
4. While the chicken is in the oven, cut the broccoli into florets and slice the stem (or use frozen). Boil in lightly salted water for 5 minutes in a saucepan. Drain the water and put on the lid to keep warm.
5. Mix all the ingredients to the garlic butter in a bowl. Set aside.
6. Serve the chicken with the broccoli and garlic butter.

Quick keto chicken garam masala

Made for: Lunch | Prep Time: 35 minutes | Servings: 04 people
Nutrition Per Servings: Kcal: 732, Protein: 33g, Fat: 65g, Net Carb: 6g

INGREDIENTS

- ❖ 1½ lbs boneless chicken thighs, sliced

- ❖ 1 red bell pepper, thinly sliced
- ❖ 3 tbsp coconut oil
- ❖ 2½ tbsp garam masala seasoning
- ❖ 2 tsp turmeric
- ❖ 2 garlic cloves, finely chopped
- ❖ 1 tsp salt
- ❖ 1¼ cups coconut cream or heavy whipping cream
- ❖ 3 tbsp fresh cilantro, roughly chopped

INSTRUCTIONS

1. Place a large skillet over medium high heat and add the coconut oil.
2. When the oil is hot, add the garam masala, turmeric and garlic into the pan. Fry for a minute while stirring, making sure it doesn't get burned.
3. Add the chicken and salt, then stir thoroughly. Fry for about 3 minutes before adding the bell pepper. Continue frying for about 2 minutes. Add the coconut cream and let it simmer, uncovered, over medium heat for 10 minutes.
4. Garnish with cilantro and serve.

Special Italian Chicken

Made for: Lunch | Prep Time: 50 minutes | Servings: 06 people
Nutrition Per Servings: Kcal: 150, Protein: 10g, Fat: 5g, Net Carb: 1g

INGREDIENTS

- ❖ 18 chicken wings, cut in halves
- ❖ 1 tablespoon turmeric
- ❖ 1 tablespoon cumin, ground
- ❖ 1 tablespoon ginger, grated
- ❖ 1 tablespoon coriander, ground
- ❖ 1 tablespoon paprika
- ❖ A pinch of cayenne pepper
- ❖ Salt and black pepper to the taste
- ❖ 2 tablespoons olive oil

- ❖ For the chutney:
- ❖ Juice of ½ lime
- ❖ 1 cup mint leaves
- ❖ 1 small ginger piece, chopped
- ❖ ¾ cup cilantro
- ❖ 1 tablespoon olive oil
- ❖ 1 tablespoon water
- ❖ Salt and black pepper to the taste 1 Serrano pepper

INSTRUCTIONS

1. In a bowl, mix 1 tablespoon ginger with cumin, coriander, paprika, turmeric, salt, pepper, cayenne and 2 tablespoons oil and stir well.
2. Add chicken wings pieces to this mix, toss to coat well and keep in the fridge for 20 minutes.

3. Heat up your grill over high heat, add marinated wings, cook for 25 minutes, turning them from time to time and transfer to a bowl.

4. In your blender, mix mint with cilantro, 1 small ginger pieces, juice from ½ lime, 1 tablespoon olive oil, salt, pepper, water and Serrano pepper and blend very well.

5. Serve your chicken wings with this sauce on the side.

Keto chicken pesto

Made for: Lunch | Prep Time: 50 minutes | Servings: 04 people
Nutrition Per Servings: Kcal: 712, Protein: 35g, Fat: 50g, Net Carb: 5g

INGREDIENTS

- ❖ 1 oz. butter
- ❖ 1½ lbs boneless, skinless boneless chicken thighs, cut into 1" (3 cm) pieces
- ❖ 1½ tsp garlic powder
- ❖ 1 cup heavy whipping cream
- ❖ 3 tbsp green pesto
- ❖ 1 lb zucchini, spiralized
- ❖ 8 oz. tomatoes, diced, or cherry tomatoes cut in half
- ❖ salt and ground black pepper, to taste

INSTRUCTIONS

1. Melt the butter in a large frying pan, over medium-high heat.
2. When the butter starts to bubble, add the garlic powder and chicken to the pan. Sauté for about 10 minutes, or until lightly browned.
3. Reduce the heat to medium-low, and add the cream and pesto. Simmer for a couple of minutes, stirring together until the mixture is creamy and well-combined.
4. Add the zucchini noodles and tomatoes. Toss to combine, and let simmer for about 2 minutes, just until the zucchini noodles become slightly tender, but still have some crispness. Season with salt and pepper to taste. Serve immediately.

Chicken and Paprika Sauce

Made for: Lunch | Prep Time: 35 minutes | Servings: 05 people
Nutrition Per Servings: Kcal: 150, Protein: 5g, Fat: 4g, Net Carb: 3g

INGREDIENTS

- ❖ 1 tablespoon coconut oil
- ❖ 3 and ½ pounds chicken breasts
- ❖ 1 cup chicken stock
- ❖ 1 and ¼ cups yellow onion, chopped
- ❖ 1 tablespoon lime juice
- ❖ ¼ cup coconut milk
- ❖ 2 teaspoons paprika
- ❖ 1 teaspoon red pepper flakes
- ❖ 2 tablespoons green onions, chopped
- ❖ Salt and black pepper to the taste

INSTRUCTIONS

1. Heat up a pan with the oil over medium high heat, add chicken, cook for 2 minutes on each side, transfer to a plate and leave aside.
2. Reduce heat to medium, add onions to the pan and cook for 4 minutes.
3. Add stock, coconut milk, pepper flakes, paprika, lime juice, salt and pepper and stir well.
4. Return chicken to the pan, add more salt and pepper, cover pan and cook for 15 minutes.
5. Divide between plates and serve.

Keto coconut salmon

Made for: Lunch | Prep Time: 35 minutes | Servings: 04 people
Nutrition Per Servings: Kcal: 765, Protein: 33g, Fat: 60g, Net Carb: 3g

INGREDIENTS

- ❖ 1¼ lbs salmon
- ❖ 1 tbsp olive oil
- ❖ 2 oz. unsweetened finely shredded coconut
- ❖ 1 tsp turmeric
- ❖ 1 tsp kosher or ground sea salt
- ❖ ½ tsp onion powder
- ❖ 4 tbsp olive oil, for frying
- ❖ 1¼ lbs Napa cabbage
- ❖ 4 oz. butter
- ❖ salt and pepper
- ❖ lemon, for serving

INSTRUCTIONS

1. Cut the salmon in 1 x 1 inch pieces. Drizzle with olive or coconut oil.
2. Mix shredded coconut, salt, turmeric and onion powder on a plate. Toss the salmon pieces in the coconut coating.
3. Fry the salmon pieces on medium high heat until golden brown. Keep warm while you prepare the cabbage.
4. Cut the cabbage in wedges and fry in butter until lightly caramelized. Season generously with salt and pepper.
5. Melt the remaining butter. Serve the salmon, cabbage and melted butter with a few wedges of fresh lemon.

Keto tuna and avocado salad

Made for: Lunch | Prep Time: 20 minutes | Servings: 04 people
Nutrition Per Servings: Kcal: 642, Protein: 41g, Fat: 45g, Net Carb: 5g

INGREDIENTS

- ❖ 24 oz. can of tuna in water
- ❖ 3 avocados, cut into eights
- ❖ 3 oz. red bell peppers, sliced
- ❖ 2 oz. red onions, sliced
- ❖ 5 oz. cucumber, quartered
- ❖ 2 oz. celery stalks, diced
- ❖ 2 tbsp lime juice
- ❖ 1/3 cup olive oil
- ❖ salt and pepper to taste

INSTRUCTIONS

1. Drain the tuna. Use a fork to flake the tuna onto a plate.
2. Slice red bell pepper and red onion into thin slices.
3. Quarter the cucumber, lengthways, remove seeds and slice.
4. Halve the celery, lengthways, and then cut into small pieces. Then peel and de-stone the avocado and cut into eighths.
5. Arrange all ingredients in layers on a large serving platter, or onto individual plates.
6. Place the lime juice and olive oil in a small jar and shake well to combine. Drizzle dressing over salad and finish off with salt and pepper to taste.

Chilli avocado

Made for: Lunch | Prep Time: 2 minutes | Servings: 01 people
Nutrition Per Servings: Kcal: 102, Protein: 1g, Fat: 10g, Net Carb: 1g

INGREDIENTS

- ❖ ½ small avocado
- ❖ ¼ tsp chilli flakes
- ❖ juice of ¼ lime

INSTRUCTIONS

1. Sprinkle the avocado with the chilli flakes, lime juice and a little black pepper, and eat with a spoon.

Keto Low-Carb Tortilla Soup

Made for: Lunch | Prep Time: 65 minutes | Servings: 04 people
Nutrition Per Servings: Kcal: 452, Protein: 25g, Fat: 35g, Net Carb: 8g

INGREDIENTS

- ❖ 1 tbsp 1 tablespoon avocado oil
- ❖ 1/2 pound rotisserie chicken, stripped the carcass of meat
- ❖ 1 whole onion, diced
- ❖ 2 cloves garlic, minced
- ❖ 1 whole carrot, peeled and diced
- ❖ 1 stalk celery, diced
- ❖ 1 cup tomatoes, diced
- ❖ 3-4 whole jalapeno peppers, diced
- ❖ 2 cups chicken stock
- ❖ 2 tsp chili powder, ground
- ❖ 1 tsp cumin powder, ground
- ❖ 1/4 tsp cayenne pepper, ground
- ❖ 1 cup full-fat cream cheese
- ❖ 1/4 cup cilantro, fresh and chopped

INSTRUCTIONS

1. Remove the chicken meat from the rotisserie chicken and put aside.
2. Heat the avocado oil in a large saucepan over medium-high heat. Saute the onion and garlic for 3 minutes until they are golden brown and softened.
3. Stir in the carrot, celery, jalapenos, tomatoes, and the stripped chicken meat. Add in all the spices and mix for 1 minute.
4. Pour in the chicken stock and bring the soup to a boil.

5. Reduce the heat to low and simmer for 20-30 minutes until the vegetables are soft and tender.
6. Stir in the heavy cream and cream cheese. Stir until cheese is melted. If the soup is too thick, add in 1/8 cup of chicken stock to make it thinner.
7. Divide the soup into 4 bowls and garnish it with chopped cilantro. Serve warm and enjoy!

Vegan Keto Green Smoothie

Made for: Lunch | Prep Time: 05 minutes | Servings: 01 people
Nutrition Per Servings: Kcal: 114, Protein: 04g, Fat:10g, Net Carb: 3g

INGREDIENTS

- ❖ 1/2 cup unsweetened almond milk
- ❖ 1/2 lemon juice
- ❖ 1 oz Avocado (about 1/8 avocado)
- ❖ 1 tbsp hemp seeds
- ❖ 1.2 tsp vanilla extract
- ❖ 1 packet keto sweetener
- ❖ 1 cup ice cubes

INSTRUCTIONS

1. Add all your ingredients except ice cubes to your blender and blend till smooth.
2. Add the ice cubes and blend some more, for about 1 minute.
3. Pour the smoothie into a glass and enjoy!
4. Pour the smoothie into a glass and enjoy!

Keto Egg Salad

Made for: Lunch | Prep Time: 10 minutes | Servings: 03 people
Nutrition Per Servings: Kcal: 443, Protein: 13g, Fat:30g, Net Carb: 6g

INGREDIENTS

- ❖ 6 Eggs Hard-boiled
- ❖ 1 Avocado Medium
- ❖ 1 tbsp Dijon mustard
- ❖ 3 tbsps Mayonnaise
- ❖ 1 tsp Lemon juice
- ❖ 1 tsp Dill Chopped (optional)
- ❖ 1 tsp Parsley Chopped (optional)

❖ Sea salt & pepper

INSTRUCTIONS

1. Break the hard-boiled eggs with the back of a fork in a large bowl. Add a pinch of salt and pepper to taste.
2. Add the ripe avocado to the bowl and mash it the fork. Sprinkle the lemon juice on top of the avocado to prevent it from browning.
3. Add mayonnaise and mustard to the egg mixture and mix until it's fully coated with the mayonnaise.
4. Sprinkle the chopped parsley and dill and serve. If you are not eating it right away, chill in the fridge.

Super Packed Cheese Omelette

Made for: Lunch | Prep Time: 15 minutes | Servings: 04 people
Nutrition Per Servings: Kcal: 438, Protein: 25g, Fat: 35g, Net Carb: 2g

INGREDIENTS

❖ 3 large mushrooms (sliced).
❖ 3 large eggs.
❖ 1 oz cheddar cheese (grated).
❖ 1 oz butter.
❖ ¼ onion (finely sliced).
❖ Pinch salt and pepper.

INSTRUCTIONS

1. In a bowl, whisk together the eggs, salt and pepper.
2. In a large frying pan, melt the butter and fry onions and mushrooms until tender.
3. Pour in the egg mixture so that it surrounds the onions and mushrooms.
4. As the sides begin to firm and it is still slightly runny in the middle, sprinkle on the cheese
5. Continue cooking until egg mixture is completely formed and cooked through.

Mediterranean sardine salad

Made for: Lunch | Prep Time: 15 minutes | Servings: 04 people
Nutrition Per Servings: Kcal: 140, Protein: 10g, Fat: 10g, Net Carb: 1g

INGREDIENTS

- ❖ 90g bag salad leaves
- ❖ handful black olives , roughly chopped
- ❖ 1 tbsp caper , drained
- ❖ 2 x 120g cans sardines in tomato sauce, drained and sauce reserved
- ❖ 1 tbsp olive oil
- ❖ 1 tbsp red wine vinegar

INSTRUCTIONS

1. Divide the salad leaves between 4 plates, then sprinkle over the olives and capers. Roughly break up the sardines and add to the salad. Mix the tomato sauce with the oil and vinegar and drizzle over the salad.

Antipasto salad

Made for: Lunch | Prep Time: 30 minutes | Servings: 02 people
Nutrition Per Servings: Kcal: 824, Protein: 38g, Fat: 65g, Net Carb: 10g

INGREDIENTS

- ❖ 10 oz. Romaine lettuce, chopped into pieces
- ❖ 2 tbsp fresh parsley, chopped
- ❖ 5 oz. fresh mozzarella cheese, sliced in small pieces
- ❖ 3 oz. Parma ham, "proscuitto", thinly sliced
- ❖ 3 oz. salami, thinly sliced
- ❖ 5 oz. canned artichokes in water, drained and quartered
- ❖ 3 oz. canned roasted red peppers, drained
- ❖ 1 oz. sun-dried tomatoes in oil, strained and chopped
- ❖ 1 oz. olives, whole and pitted, or sliced
- ❖ 1/3 cup fresh basil
- ❖ 1 red chili pepper, finely chopped
- ❖ ½ tbsp sea salt
- ❖ 4 tbsp olive oil

INSTRUCTIONS

1. Chop or tear the lettuce into smaller pieces. Distribute it on plates or a large platter. Add the parsley.
2. Layer the antipasto ingredients on top.
3. In a mortar or small bowl, add basil, finely chopped chili, and salt. Crush with a wooden spoon or use the mortar and pestle. Sprinkle over salad and drizzle with olive oil.

Italian keto plate

Made for: Lunch | Prep Time: 05 minutes | Servings: 02 people
Nutrition Per Servings: Kcal: 824, Protein: 38g, Fat: 65g, Net Carb: 10g

INGREDIENTS

- ❖ 7 oz. fresh mozzarella cheese
- ❖ 7 oz. prosciutto, sliced
- ❖ 2 tomatoes
- ❖ 1⁄3 cup olive oil
- ❖ 10 green olives
- ❖ salt and pepper

INSTRUCTIONS

1. Put tomatoes, prosciutto, cheese and olives on a plate. Serve with olive oil and season with salt and pepper to taste.

Low-carb baked eggs

Made for: Lunch | Prep Time: 15 minutes | Servings: 01 people
Nutrition Per Servings: Kcal: 498, Protein: 41g, Fat: 35g, Net Carb: 2g

INGREDIENTS

- ❖ 3 oz. ground beef or ground lamb or ground pork, use left-overs or cook it any way you like. You can also use this recipe.
- ❖ 2 eggs
- ❖ 2 oz. shredded cheese

INSTRUCTIONS

1. Preheat the oven to 400°F (200°C).
2. Arrange cooked ground-beef mixture in a small baking dish. Then make two holes with a spoon and crack the eggs into them.
3. Sprinkle shredded cheese on top.
4. Bake in the oven until the eggs are done, about 10-15 minutes.
5. Let cool for a while. The eggs and ground meat get very hot!

Keto crab meat and egg plate

Made for: Lunch | Prep Time: 15 minutes | Servings: 02 people
Nutrition Per Servings: Kcal: 498, Protein: 41g, Fat: 35g, Net Carb: 2g

INGREDIENTS

- ❖ 4 eggs
- ❖ 12 oz. canned crab meat
- ❖ 2 avocados
- ❖ ½ cup cottage cheese
- ❖ ½ cup mayonnaise
- ❖ 1½ oz. baby spinach
- ❖ 2 tbsp olive oil
- ❖ ½ tsp chili flakes (optional)
- ❖ salt and pepper

INSTRUCTIONS

1. Begin by cooking the eggs. Lower them carefully into boiling water and boil for 4-8 minutes depending on whether you like them soft or hard boiled.
2. Cool the eggs in ice-cold water for 1-2 minutes when they're done; this will make it easier to remove the shell. Peel eggs.
3. Place eggs, crab meat, avocado, cottage cheese, mayonnaise and spinach on a plate.
4. Drizzle olive oil over the spinach. Season with salt and pepper. Sprinkle optional chili flakes on the avocado and serve.

Keto mackerel and egg plate

Made for: Lunch | Prep Time: 15 minutes | Servings: 02 people
Nutrition Per Servings: Kcal: 689, Protein: 35g, Fat: 60g, Net Carb: 4g

INGREDIENTS

- ❖ 4 eggs
- ❖ 2 tbsp butter for frying
- ❖ 8 oz. canned mackerel in tomato sauce
- ❖ 2 oz. lettuce
- ❖ ½ red onion
- ❖ ¼ cup olive oil
- ❖ salt and pepper

INSTRUCTIONS

1. Fry the eggs in butter, just the way you want them – sunny side up or over easy.
2. Put lettuce, thin slices of red onion and mackerel on a plate together with the eggs. Season to taste with salt and pepper. Drizzle olive oil over the salad and serve.

Keto bacon and eggs plate

Made for: Lunch | Prep Time: 15 minutes | Servings: 02 people
Nutrition Per Servings: Kcal: 974, Protein: 27g, Fat: 90g, Net Carb: 8g

INGREDIENTS

- ❖ 5 oz. bacon
- ❖ 4 eggs
- ❖ 2 avocados
- ❖ 1 oz. walnuts
- ❖ 1 green bell pepper
- ❖ salt and pepper
- ❖ 1 tbsp fresh chives, finely chopped (optional)

Serving
- ❖ 1 oz. arugula lettuce
- ❖ 2 tbsp olive oil

INSTRUCTIONS

1. Fry the bacon over medium heat until crispy.
2. Remove from pan and keep warm. Leave the fat that's accumulated in the pan. Lower the heat to medium low and fry the eggs in the same frying pan.
3. Place bacon, eggs, avocado, nuts, bell pepper and arugula on a plate.
4. Drizzle the remaining bacon fat on top of the eggs. Season to taste.

Keto halloumi cheese and avocado plate

Made for: Lunch | Prep Time: 15 minutes | Servings: 02 people
Nutrition Per Servings: Kcal: 1112, Protein: 36g, Fat: 99g, Net Carb: 12g

INGREDIENTS

- ❖ 10 oz. halloumi cheese
- ❖ 2 tbsp butter for frying
- ❖ 2 avocados

- ❖ ¼ cucumber
- ❖ 1/3 cup sour cream
- ❖ 2 tbsp olive oil
- ❖ ¼ lemon (optional)
- ❖ 2 tbsp pistachio nuts
- ❖ salt and pepper

INSTRUCTIONS

1. Slice the cheese into serving-sized portions and fry it in butter over medium heat until it becomes golden. A few minutes on each side should be about right.
2. Serve with avocado, cucumber, sour cream, pistachios and lemon.
3. Drizzle olive oil over the vegetables. Season with salt and pepper.

Keto cauliflower hash with eggs

Made for: Lunch | Prep Time: 25 minutes | Servings: 04 people
Nutrition Per Servings: Kcal: 890, Protein: 16g, Fat: 85g, Net Carb: 9g

INGREDIENTS

- ❖ 1 lb grated cauliflower
- ❖ 3 oz. butter
- ❖ salt and pepper
- ❖ 4 eggs
- ❖ 3 oz. pimientos de padron or poblano peppers
- ❖ 1 tsp olive oil
- ❖ ½ cup mayonnaise
- ❖ 1 tsp garlic powder or onion powder (optional)

INSTRUCTIONS

1. Mix mayonnaise and garlic or onion powder in a small bowl and set aside.
2. Grate the cauliflower, including the stem; either use a grater or chop into rough but fairly small pieces in a food processor.
3. Fry grated cauliflower for about five minutes in a generous amount of butter or oil. Season with salt and pepper to taste.
4. Brush some oil on the poblanos. Fry or grill until the skin starts to bubble a little bit.
5. Fry the eggs as you like them. Season with salt and pepper to taste. Serve directly with the roasted poblanos and cauliflower hash. Top with a nice dollop of the seasoned mayo.

Delicious Broccoli Soup

Made for: Lunch | Prep Time: 45 minutes | Servings: 04 people
Nutrition Per Servings: Kcal: 352, Protein: 10g, Fat: 30g, Net Carb: 6g

INGREDIENTS

- ❖ 1 white onion, chopped
- ❖ 1 tablespoon ghee
- ❖ 2 cups veggie stock
- ❖ Salt and black pepper to the taste
- ❖ 2 cups water
- ❖ 2 garlic cloves, minced
- ❖ 1 cup heavy cream
- ❖ 8 ounces cheddar cheese, grated
- ❖ 12 ounces broccoli florets ½ teaspoon paprika

INSTRUCTIONS

1. Heat up a pot with the ghee over medium heat, add onion and garlic, stir and cook for 5 minutes.
2. Add stock, cream, water, salt, pepper and paprika, stir and bring to a boil.
3. Add broccoli, stir and simmer soup for 25 minutes.
4. Transfer to your food processor and blend well.
5. Add cheese and blend again.
6. Divide into soup bowls and serve hot.

Keto falafels

Made for: Lunch | Prep Time: 50 minutes | Servings: 04 people
Nutrition Per Servings: Kcal: 580, Protein: 30g, Fat: 46g, Net Carb: 6g

INGREDIENTS

- ❖ 8 oz. mushrooms, sliced
- ❖ ½ cup light olive oil, divided
- ❖ ½ cup pumpkin seeds
- ❖ ½ cup almonds
- ❖ ¾ cup vegan unflavored protein powder (pea protein)
- ❖ ¼ cup water
- ❖ 4 tbsp chia seeds
- ❖ 2 garlic cloves, minced
- ❖ 2 tbsp fresh parsley, finely chopped
- ❖ 1 tsp salt
- ❖ 1 tsp onion powder
- ❖ 1 tsp ground cumin
- ❖ 1 tsp ground coriander seed

* ❖ ¼ tsp ground black pepper

INSTRUCTIONS

1. Preheat the oven to 350°F (175°C).
2. Heat a large dry frying pan and roast the almonds and pumpkin seeds until lightly browned and fragrant. Put them in a food processor and pulse for a couple of minutes.
3. Fry the mushrooms in a large frying pan in ⅓ of the olive oil until soft and moist. Add the mushrooms, and the remaining oil to the food processor, together with the rest of the ingredients. Mix for a couple of minutes. Let sit for about 5 minutes.
4. Shape the mixture into 1½ inch (4 cm) balls. Place the balls on a baking sheet.
5. Bake in the oven for 20 minutes or until crispy. Serve warm, together with the side dish of your choice.

Prosciutto-wrapped salmon skewers

Made for: Lunch | Prep Time: 35 minutes | Servings: 04 people
Nutrition Per Servings: Kcal: 678, Protein: 30g, Fat: 60g, Net Carb: 1g

INGREDIENTS

* ❖ Salmon skewers
* ❖ ¼ cup fresh basil, finely chopped
* ❖ 1 lb salmon, frozen in pieces
* ❖ 1 pinch ground black pepper
* ❖ 3½ oz. prosciutto, in slices
* ❖ 1 tbsp olive oil
* ❖ 8 wooden skewers

Serving
* ❖ 1 cup mayonnaise

INSTRUCTIONS

1. Soak the skewers.
2. Chop the basil finely with a sharp knife.
3. Cut the almost thawed lax-filet pieces length-wise and mount on the skewers.
4. Roll the skewers in the chopped basil and pepper.
5. Slice the prosciutto into thin strips and wrap around the salmon.
6. Cover in olive oil and fry in a pan, oven or on the grill.

7.   Serve with the mayonnaise or a hearty salad and a rich aioli.

Simple Lunch Apple Salad

Made for: Lunch | Prep Time: 50 minutes | Servings: 04 people
Nutrition Per Servings: Kcal: 678, Protein: 30g, Fat: 60g, Net Carb: 1g

INGREDIENTS

- ❖ 2 cups broccoli florets, roughly chopped
- ❖ 2 ounces pecans, chopped
- ❖ 1 apple, cored and grated
- ❖ 1 green onion stalk, finely chopped
- ❖ Salt and black pepper to the taste
- ❖ 2 teaspoons poppy seeds
- ❖ 1 teaspoon apple cider vinegar
- ❖ ¼ cup mayonnaise
- ❖ ½ teaspoon lemon juice ¼ cup sour cream

INSTRUCTIONS

1.   In a salad bowl, mix apple with broccoli, green onion and pecans and stir.
2.   Add poppy seeds, salt and pepper and toss gently.
3.   In a bowl, mix mayo with sour cream, vinegar and lemon juice and whisk well.
4.   Pour this over salad, toss to coat well and serve cold for lunch!

Crab-stuffed avocados

Made for: Lunch | Prep Time: 10 minutes | Servings: 04 people
Nutrition Per Servings: Kcal: 204, Protein: 06g, Fat: 19g, Net Carb: 2g

INGREDIENTS

- ❖ 100g white crabmeat
- ❖ 1 tsp Dijon mustard
- ❖ 2 tbsp olive oil
- ❖ handful basil leaves, shredded with a few of the smaller leaves left whole, to serve
- ❖ 1 red chilli , deseeded and chopped
- ❖ 2 avocados

INSTRUCTIONS

1. To make the crab mix, flake the crabmeat into a small bowl and mix in the mustard and oil, then season to taste. Can be made the day ahead. Add the basil and chilli just before serving.
2. To serve, halve and stone the avocados. Fill each cavity with a quarter of the crab mix, scatter with a few of the smaller basil leaves and eat with teaspoons.

Salmon, avocado & cucumber salad

Made for: Lunch | Prep Time: 18 minutes | Servings: 04 people
Nutrition Per Servings: Kcal: 458, Protein: 23g, Fat: 40g, Net Carb: 7g

INGREDIENTS

- ❖ 4 skinless salmon fillets , approx 100g each
- ❖ 3 avocados
- ❖ 1 cucumber
- ❖ 400g bag mixed salad leaves
- ❖ For the dressing
- ❖ 4 tbsp chopped mint
- ❖ grated zest 1 and juice o limes
- ❖ 2 tsp clear honey
- ❖ 3 tbsp olive oil , plus a little extra for the salmon

INSTRUCTIONS

1. Season the salmon, then rub with oil. Mix the dressing ingredients together. Halve, stone, peel and slice the avocados. Halve and quarter the cucumber lengthways, then cut into slices. Divide salad, avocado and cucumber between four plates, then drizzle with half the dressing.
2. Heat a non-stick pan. Add the salmon and fry for 3-4 mins on each side until crisp but still moist inside. Put a salmon fillet on top of each salad and drizzle over the remaining dressing. Serve warm.

Asparagus, pea & feta frittata

Made for: Lunch | Prep Time: 27 minutes | Servings: 02 people
Nutrition Per Servings: Kcal: 309, Protein: 18g, Fat: 23g, Net Carb: 7g

INGREDIENTS

- ❖ 1 tbsp olive oil
- ❖ ½ bunch asparagus spears (save the rest for Rosti fish cakes, see 'goes well with'), trimmed and cut into 5cm pieces

- 100g frozen petits pois or peas
- 50g feta cheese
- 1 tbsp freshly chopped mint
- 3 large eggs , beaten
- 1 tbsp balsamic vinegar glaze or balsamic vinegar
- leftover roast cherry tomatoes (from Bacon, tomato & broccoli pasta, see 'goes well with')
- crisp green salad , to serve

INSTRUCTIONS

1. Heat oven to 180C/160C fan/gas 4. Put the olive oil in a small (about 600ml) shallow ovenproof dish. Place in the oven to heat for 2-3 mins, add the asparagus and peas to the hot oil and gently toss to coat. Return to the oven for 2 mins, then remove from the oven and crumble over the feta.
2. Meanwhile, beat the mint into the eggs and season well with lots of ground black pepper. Remove the dish from the oven and pour over the eggs, then bake for 15 mins until the eggs have set.
3. Meanwhile, drizzle the balsamic glaze or vinegar over the leftover roast tomatoes. Serve the frittata with the balsamic tomatoes and a crisp green salad.

Dinner Recipes

Baked Eggs and Zoodles

Made for: Dinner | Prep Time: 25 minutes | Servings: 02 people
Nutrition Per Servings: Kcal: 633, Protein: 20g, Fat: 53g, Net Carb: 20g

INGREDIENTS

- Nonstick spray
- 3 zucchini, spiralized into noodles
- 2 tablespoons extra-virgin olive oil
- Kosher salt and freshly ground black pepper

- 4 large eggs
- Red-pepper flakes, for garnishing
- Fresh basil, for garnishing
- 2 avocados, halved and thinly sliced

INSTRUCTIONS

1. Preheat the oven to 350°F. Lightly grease a baking sheet with nonstick spray.
2. In a large bowl, toss the zucchini noodles and olive oil to combine. Season with salt and pepper. Divide into 4 even portions, transfer to the baking sheet and shape each into a nest.
3. Gently crack an egg into the center of each nest. Bake until the eggs are set, 9 to 11 minutes. Season with salt and pepper; garnish with red-pepper flakes and basil. Serve alongside the avocado slices.

Fried Chicken Recipe

Made for: Dinner | Prep Time: 50 minutes | Servings: 01 people
Nutrition Per Servings: Kcal: 308, Protein: 40g, Fat: 14g, Net Carb: 1g

INGREDIENTS

- 4 oz pork rinds
- 1.5 tsp thyme dried
- 1 tsp sea salt dried
- 1 tsp black pepper dried
- 1 tsp oregano dried
- 0.5 tsp garlic powder dried
- 1 tsp smoked paprika dried

- 12 legs and thighs bone-in chicken skinless, medium-size pieces
- 1 egg
- 2 oz mayonnaise
- 3 tbsp Dijon mustard

1. Preheat oven to 400 degrees Fahrenheit.
2. Crush pork rinds into a powder-like texture, leaving in a few larger pieces.
3. Combine pork rinds with thyme, salt, pepper, oregano, garlic powder, and smoked paprika. Spread out into a thin layer on a large plate or flat dish.
4. In a wide bowl, combine egg, mayo, and Dijon mustard. Dip each piece of chicken into the egg-mayo mixture, then roll in the pork rind mixture until evenly coated.
5. Place chicken on a wire rack over a baking sheet and bake for 40 minutes.

Buffalo Chicken Strips

Made for: Dinner | Prep Time: 25 minutes | Servings: 03 people
Nutrition Per Servings: 683 Calories, 54g Fats, 4.8g Net Carbs, and 41g Protein

INGREDIENTS

- ❖ 5 Chicken Breasts Pounded to 1/2" Thickness
- ❖ 3/4 Cup Almond Flour
- ❖ 1/2 Cup Hot Sauce
- ❖ 1/4 Cup Olive Oil
- ❖ 3 Tbsp. Butter
- ❖ 3 Tbsp. Blue Cheese Crumbles

- ❖ 2 Large Eggs
- ❖ 1 Tbsp. Paprika
- ❖ 1 Tbsp. Chili powder
- ❖ 2 tsp. Salt
- ❖ 2 tsp. Pepper
- ❖ 1 tsp. Garlic Powder
- ❖ 1 tsp. Onion Powder

INSTRUCTIONS

1. Preheat oven to 400F.
2. In a ramekin, combine paprika, chili powder, salt, pepper, garlic powder, and onion powder.
3. Pound out chicken breasts to 1/2" thickness, then cut the chicken breasts in half.
4. Sprinkle 1/3 of the spice mix over the chicken breast, then flip them over and do the same with 1/3 of the spice mix.
5. In a bowl, combine almond flour and 1/3 of the spice mix.
6. In another container, crack 2 eggs and whisk them.
7. Dip each piece of seasoned chicken into the spice mix and then into the almond flour. Make sure each side is coated well.
8. Lay each piece on a cooling rack on top of a foiled baking sheet.
9. Bake the chicken for 15 minutes.
10. Take the chicken out of the oven and turn your oven to broil. Drizzle 2 Tbsp. olive oil over the chicken.

11. Broil for 5 minutes, flip the breasts, drizzle with remaining olive oil, and broil again for 5 minutes.
12. In a sauce pan, combined 1/2 Cup of hot sauce with 3 Tbsp. butter.
13. Serve chicken with slathering of hot sauce and blue cheese crumbles.

Cheddar Chorizo Meatballs

Made for: Dinner | Prep Time: 40 minutes | Servings: 24 people
Nutrition Per Servings: 115 Calories, 7.8g Fats, 0.8g Net Carbs, and 9.9g Protein.

INGREDIENTS

- 1 1/2 lb. Ground Beef
- 1 1/2 Chorizo Sausages
- 1 Cup Cheddar Cheese
- 1 Cup Tomato Sauce
- 1/3 Cup Crushed Pork Rinds

- 2 Large Eggs
- 1 tsp. Cumin
- 1 tsp. Chili Powder
- 1 tsp. Kosher Salt

INSTRUCTIONS

1. Preheat oven to 350F.
2. Break up sausage into small pieces so that it will mix well with the ground beef.
3. Add your ground beef, ground pork rinds, spices, chee-se, and eggs to the sausage.
4. Mix everything together well until you can form meat-balls.
5. Roll your meatballs out into circles and place them in a foiled baking tray.
6. Bake in the oven for 30-35 minutes, or until meatballs are cooked through.
7. Spoon tomato sauce over meatballs and serve.

Tangy & Tasty BBQ Pork Ribs

Made for: Dinner | Prep Time: 30 minutes | Servings: 2 people
Nutrition Per Servings: 1000 Calories, 55.5g Fats, 85g Net Carbs, and 6g Protein.

INGREDIENTS

- 48 oz pork ribs.
- ¼ cup dijon mustard.
- 4 tbsp paprika powder.
- 2 tbsp butter.
- 2 tbsp apple cider vinegar.
- 2 tbsp garlic powder.
- 1 ½ tbsp black pepper.
- 1 tbsp salt.

- 1 tbsp chilli powder.
- 2 tsp onion powder.

INSTRUCTIONS

1. Preheat oven at 400 degrees.
2. In a bowl, mix mustard and vinegar.
3. In a separate bowl, mix paprika, garlic, pepper, salt, chilli, and onion powder.
4. Have a large sheet of foil next to both bowls. Dip each rib into the vinegar mixture (ensure both sides are covered) then dip into the spice mixture (provide bones are completely covered)—place ribs on the foil.
5. Add the butter to the top of the ribs. Wrap the ribs in foil (use another piece to secure).
6. Place ribs on a baking tray and bake for 60 minutes.
7. When ribs are ready, remove from oven and foil.
8. Grill on high heat to give additional colour.

Keto chicken enchilada bowl

Made for: Dinner | Prep Time: 30 minutes | Servings: 4 people
Nutrition Per Servings: Kcal: 568, Protein: 38g, Fat: 40g, Net Carb: 6g

INGREDIENTS

- ❖ Two tablespoon coconut oil (for searing chicken)
- ❖ 1 pound of boneless, skinless chicken thighs
- ❖ 3/4 cup red enchilada sauce (recipe from Low Carb Maven)
- ❖ 1/4 cup water
- ❖ 1/4 cup chopped onion
- ❖ 1– 4 oz can dice green chiles

INSTRUCTIONS

1. In a pot or dutch oven over medium heat, melt the coconut oil. Once hot, sear chicken thighs until lightly brown.
2. Pour in enchilada sauce and water, then add onion and green chiles. Reduce heat to a simmer and cover. Cook chicken for 17-25 minutes or until chicken is tender and fully cooked through to at least 165 degrees internal temperature.
3. Carefully removes the chicken and place it onto a work surface. Chop or shred chicken (your preference), then add it back into the pot. Let the chicken simmer uncovered for an additional 10 minutes to absorb flavour and allow the sauce to reduce a little.
4. To serve, top with avocado, cheese, jalapeno, sour cream, tomato, and any other desired toppings. Feel free to customize these to your preference. Serve alone or over cauliflower rice, if desired, just be sure to update your nutrition info as needed.

Chicken and Snap

Made for: Dinner | Prep Time: 30 minutes | Servings: 4 people
Nutrition Per Servings: Kcal: 221, Protein: 20g, Fat: 25g, Net Carb: 4g

INGREDIENTS

- ❖ Two tablespoons vegetable oil
- ❖ One bunch scallions, thinly sliced
- ❖ Two garlic cloves, minced
- ❖ One red bell pepper, thinly sliced
- ❖ 2½ cups snap peas
- ❖ 1¼ cups boneless skinless chicken breast, thinly sliced
- ❖ Salt and freshly ground Black Pepper
- ❖ Three tablespoons soy sauce
- ❖ Two tablespoons rice vinegar
- ❖ Two teaspoons Sriracha (optional)
- ❖ Two tablespoons sesame seeds, plus more for finishing
- ❖ Three tablespoons chopped fresh cilantro, plus more for finishing

INSTRUCTIONS

1. In a large sauté pan, heat the oil over medium heat. Add the scallions and garlic, and sauté until fragrant, about 1 minute. Add the bell pepper and snap peas and sauté until just tender, 2 to 3 minutes.
2. Add the chicken and cook until it is golden and fully cooked, and the vegetables are tender 4 to 5 minutes.
3. Add the soy sauce, rice vinegar, Sriracha (if using), and sesame seeds; toss well to combine. Allow the mixture to simmer for 1 to 2 minutes. Stir in the cilantro, then garnish with a sprinkle of extra cilantro and sesame seeds. Serve immediately.

Keto chicken casserole

Made for: Dinner | Prep Time: 65 minutes | Servings: 6 people
Nutrition Per Servings: Kcal: 740, Protein: 36g, Fat: 60g, Net Carb: 6g

INGREDIENTS

- ❖ ¾ cup heavy whipping cream or sour cream
- ❖ ½ cup cream cheese
- ❖ 3 tbsp green pesto

- ❖ ½ lemon, the juice
- ❖ salt and pepper
- ❖ 1½ oz. butter

- ❖ 2 lbs skinless boneless chicken thighs, cut into bite-sized pieces
- ❖ 1 leek, finely chopped
- ❖ 4 oz. cherry tomatoes, halved
- ❖ 1 lb cauliflower, cut into small florets
- ❖ 7 oz. shredded cheese

INSTRUCTIONS

1. Preheat the oven to 400°F (200°C).
2. Mix cream and cream cheese with pesto and lemon juice. Salt and pepper to taste.
3. In a large pan over medium high heat, melt the butter. Add the chicken, season with salt and pepper, and fry until they turn a nice golden brown.
4. Place the chicken in a greased 9 x 13 inch (23 x 33 cm) baking dish, and pour in the cream mixture.
5. Top chicken with leek, tomatoes and cauliflower.
6. Sprinkle cheese on top and bake in the middle of the oven for at least 30 minutes or until the chicken is fully cooked. If the casserole is at risk of burning before it's done, cover it with a piece of aluminium foil, lower the heat and let cook for a little longer.

Chicken Wings

Made for: Dinner | Prep Time: 35 minutes | Servings: 4 people
Nutrition Per Servings: Kcal: 420, Protein: 10g, Fat: 20g, Net Carb: 2g

INGREDIENTS

- ❖ ¼ cup olive oil
- ❖ 1 red onion, chopped
- ❖ 4 chicken breasts, skinless and boneless
- ❖ 4 garlic cloves, minced
- ❖ Salt and black pepper to the taste
- ❖ ½ cup Italian olives, pitted and chopped
- ❖ 4 anchovy fillets, chopped
- ❖ 1 tablespoon capers, chopped
- ❖ 1 pound tomatoes, chopped ½ teaspoon red chili flakes

INSTRUCTIONS

1. Season chicken with salt and pepper and rub with half of the oil.
2. Place into a pan which you've heated over high temperature, cook for 2 minutes, flip and cook for 2 minutes more.
3. Introduce chicken breasts in the oven at 450 degrees F and bake for 8 minutes.
4. Take chicken out of the oven and divide between plates.
5. Heat up the same pan with the rest of the oil over medium heat, add capers, onion, garlic, olives, anchovies, chili flakes and capers, stir and cook for 1 minute.
6. Add salt, pepper and tomatoes, stir and cook for 2 minutes more.
7. Drizzle this over chicken breasts and serve

Chicken salad with guacamole

Made for: Dinner | Prep Time: 40 minutes | Servings: 2 people
Nutrition Per Servings: Kcal: 912, Protein: 81g, Fat: 50g, Net Carb: 21g

INGREDIENTS

Cajun spice mix

- ❖ 4 tsp sweet paprika powder
- ❖ 3 tbsp dried thyme
- ❖ 2 garlic cloves, minced
- ❖ 1 pinch cayenne pepper
- ❖ 1 tbsp olive oil
- ❖ 1 lb chicken breasts (without skin)
- ❖ 7 oz. sugar snap peas

- ❖ 4 tomatoes
- ❖ 3 tbsp olive oil
- ❖ salt and ground black pepper
- ❖ 1 avocado
- ❖ 1 lime, the juice
- ❖ 2 oz. arugula lettuce

INSTRUCTIONS

1. In a bowl, make the Cajun spice mix. Combine the paprika, thyme, garlic, cayenne, and olive oil. Cut the chicken into long strips. Add the chicken and coat with the spice mixture. Let the chicken marinate for at least 5 minutes (see tip).
2. Bring a saucepan of water to a boil. Add the peas and cook until al dente. Drain well.
3. Quarter, core, and seed the tomatoes. Slice the tomatoes into thin wedges. Do this over a sieve and keep the juices for the vinaigrette.
4. Make a vinaigrette with the tomato juice, 2/3 of the olive oil, and salt and pepper.
5. Halve, pit, and peel the avocado; put the flesh in a bowl and add the lime juice. Season with salt and pepper, and mash.
6. In a skillet over medium heat, cook the chicken in the rest of the olive oil for 10 to 15 minutes, until cooked through.
7. Toss the tomatoes and peas with the arugula, and arrange them on plates.
8. Divide the guacamole and chicken strips between the plates. Serve the vinaigrette separately.

Buffalo drumsticks with chili aioli

Made for: Dinner | Prep Time: 55 minutes | Servings: 4 people
Nutrition Per Servings: Kcal: 572, Protein: 35g, Fat: 40g, Net Carb: 2g

INGREDIENTS

- Chili aioli
- 1⁄3 cup mayonnaise
- 1 tbsp smoked paprika powder or smoked chili powder
- 1 garlic clove, minced
- 2 lbs chicken drumsticks or chicken wings
- 2 tbsp olive oil or coconut oil

- 2 tbsp white wine vinegar
- 1 tbsp tomato paste
- 1 tsp salt
- 1 tsp paprika powder
- 1 tbsp tabasco
- butter or olive oil, for greasing the baking dish

INSTRUCTIONS

1. Preheat the oven to 450° (220°C).
2. Put the drumsticks in a plastic bag.
3. Mix the ingredients for the marinade in a small bowl and pour into the plastic bag. Shake the bag thoroughly and let marinate for 10 minutes in room temperature.
4. Coat a baking dish with oil. Place the drumsticks in the baking dish and let bake for 30–40 minutes or until they are done and have turned a nice color.
5. Mix together mayonnaise, garlic and chili.

Keto grilled tuna salad

Made for: Dinner | Prep Time: 35 minutes | Servings: 2 people
Nutrition Per Servings: Kcal: 975, Protein: 55g, Fat: 84g, Net Carb: 7g

INGREDIENTS

- 2 eggs
- 8 oz. green asparagus
- 1 tbsp olive oil
- ¾ lb fresh tuna, in slices
- ¼ lb leafy greens
- 2 oz. cherry tomatoes
- ½ red onion

- 2 tbsp pumpkin seeds
- salt and pepper
- Garlic dressing
- 2⁄3 cup mayonnaise
- 2 tbsp water
- 2 tsp garlic powder
- salt and pepper

INSTRUCTIONS

1. Combine ingredients for the garlic dressing. Set aside.
2. Place the eggs in boiling water for 7-10 minutes. Cool in ice water for easier peeling.
3. Cut the asparagus into lengths and quickly fry in a hot pan without oil or butter. Set aside.
4. Brush the tuna with oil and fry or grill for a few minutes on each side. Season with salt and pepper generously.

5. Add leafy greens, asparagus, peeled eggs cut in halves, tomatoes and thinly sliced onion to a plate.

6. Slice the tuna and distribute evenly over the salad. Pour over the dressing and sprinkle with pumpkin seeds.

Keto pimiento cheese meatballs

Made for: Dinner | Prep Time: 40 minutes | Servings: 4 people
Nutrition Per Servings: Kcal: 652, Protein: 40g, Fat: 51g, Net Carb: 1g

INGREDIENTS

Pimiento cheese

- ❖ 1/3 cup mayonnaise
- ❖ ¼ cup pimientos or pickled jalapeños
- ❖ 1 tsp paprika powder or chili powder
- ❖ 1 tbsp Dijon mustard
- ❖ 1 pinch cayenne pepper
- ❖ 4 oz. cheddar cheese, grated

Meatballs

- ❖ 1½ lbs ground beef
- ❖ 1 egg
- ❖ salt and pepper
- ❖ 2 tbsp butter, for frying

INSTRUCTIONS

1. Start by mixing all ingredients for the pimiento cheese in a large bowl.

2. Add ground beef and the egg to the cheese mixture. Use a wooden spoon or clean hands to combine. Salt and pepper to taste.

3. Form large meatballs and fry them in butter or oil in a skillet on medium heat until they are thoroughly cooked.

4. Serve with a side dish of your choice, a green salad and perhaps a homemade mayonnaise.

Unbelievable Chicken Dish

Made for: Dinner | Prep Time: 60 minutes | Servings: 4 people
Nutrition Per Servings: Kcal: 457, Protein: 57g, Fat: 20g, Net Carb: 2g

INGREDIENTS

- ❖ 3 pounds chicken breasts
- ❖ 2 ounces muenster cheese, cubed
- ❖ 2 ounces cream cheese
- ❖ 4 ounces cheddar cheese, cubed
- ❖ 2 ounces provolone cheese, cubed
- ❖ 1 zucchini, shredded
- ❖ Salt and black pepper to the taste
- ❖ 1 teaspoon garlic, minced
- ❖ ½ cup bacon, cooked and crumbled

INSTRUCTIONS

1. Season zucchini with salt and pepper, leave aside few minutes, squeeze well and transfer to a bowl.
2. Add bacon, garlic, more salt and pepper, cream cheese, cheddar cheese, muenster cheese and provolone cheese and stir.
3. Cut slits into chicken breasts, season with salt and pepper and stuff with zucchini and cheese mix.
4. Place on a lined baking sheet, introduce in the oven at 400 degrees F and bake for 45 minutes.
5. Divide between plates and serve.

Keto ground beef and green beans

Made for: Dinner | Prep Time: 30 minutes | Servings: 2 people
Nutrition Per Servings: Kcal: 698, Protein: 35g, Fat: 60g, Net Carb: 5g

INGREDIENTS

- ❖ 10 oz. ground beef
- ❖ 9 oz. fresh green beans
- ❖ 3½ oz. butter
- ❖ salt and pepper
- ❖ 1/3 cup mayonnaise or crème fraîche (optional)

INSTRUCTIONS

1. Rinse and trim the green beans.
2. Heat up a generous dollop of butter in a frying pan where you can fit both the ground beef and the green beans.
3. Brown the ground beef on high heat until it's almost done. Add salt and pepper.
4. Lower the heat somewhat. Add more butter and fry the beans for 5 minutes in the same pan. Stir the ground beef every now and then.
5. Season beans with salt and pepper. Serve with remaining butter and add mayonnaise or crème fraiche if you need more fat for satiety.

Italian keto meatballs

Made for: Dinner | Prep Time: 50 minutes | Servings: 4 people
Nutrition Per Servings: Kcal: 623, Protein: 40g, Fat: 50g, Net Carb: 4g

INGREDIENTS

- ❖ 1 lb ground beef
- ❖ 2 oz. parmesan cheese, grated
- ❖ 1 egg
- ❖ 1 tsp salt
- ❖ ½ tbsp dried basil
- ❖ ½ tsp onion powder
- ❖ 1 tsp garlic powder
- ❖ ½ tsp ground black pepper

- ❖ 3 tbsp olive oil
- ❖ 14 oz. canned whole tomatoes
- ❖ 2 tbsp fresh parsley, finely chopped
- ❖ 7 oz. fresh spinach
- ❖ 2 oz. butter
- ❖ 5 oz. fresh mozzarella cheese ball
- ❖ salt and pepper

INSTRUCTIONS

1. Place ground beef, parmesan cheese, egg, salt and spices in a bowl and blend thoroughly. Form the mixture into meatballs, about 1 oz (30 grams) each. It helps to keep your hands wet while forming the balls.
2. Heat up the olive oil in a large skillet and sauté the meatballs until they're golden brown on all sides.
3. Lower the heat and add the canned tomatoes. Let simmer for 15 minutes, stirring every couple of minutes. Season with salt and pepper to taste. Add parsley and stir. You can prepare the dish up to this point for freezing.
4. Melt the butter in a separate frying pan and fry the spinach for 1-2 minutes, stirring continuously. Season with salt and pepper to taste. Add the spinach to the meatballs, and stir to combine.
5. Serve with mozzarella cheese on top, torn into bite-sized pieces.

Italian cabbage stir-fry

Made for: Dinner | Prep Time: 45 minutes | Servings: 4 people
Nutrition Per Servings: Kcal: 969, Protein: 35g, Fat: 87g, Net Carb: 8g

INGREDIENTS

- ❖ 1½ lbs green cabbage
- ❖ 5 oz. butter, divided
- ❖ 1¼ lbs ground beef
- ❖ 1 tbsp white wine vinegar
- ❖ 1 tsp salt
- ❖ 1 tsp onion powder
- ❖ ¼ tsp pepper

- ❖ 2 tbsp tomato paste
- ❖ 2 garlic cloves, finely chopped
- ❖ 3 oz. leeks, thinly sliced
- ❖ 1 oz. fresh basil, chopped
- ❖ 1 cup mayonnaise or sour cream, for serving

INSTRUCTIONS

1. Shred the green cabbage finely with a sharp knife or in a food processor.
2. In a large frying pan, over medium heat, melt half of the butter. Add the cabbage and fry for about 10 minutes, or until just softened.
3. Add vinegar, salt, onion powder, and pepper. Stir and fry for 2-3 minutes, or until well incorporated. Transfer the sauteed cabbage to a large bowl.
4. Heat the rest of the butter in the pan. Add the garlic and leeks, and sauté for a minute.
5. Add meat, and continue frying until cooked through. Sauté until most of the liquid has evaporated.
6. Add tomato paste and mix well. Lower the heat a little and add reserved cabbage and fresh basil. Stir until cooked through.
7. Adjust seasoning and serve with a dollop of sour cream or mayonnaise.

Delicious Crusted Chicken

Made for: Dinner | Prep Time: 50 minutes | Servings: 4 people
Nutrition Per Servings: Kcal: 402, Protein: 46g, Fat: 23g, Net Carb: 1g

INGREDIENTS

- ❖ 4 bacon slices, cooked and crumbled
- ❖ 4 chicken breasts, skinless and boneless
- ❖ 1 tablespoon water
- ❖ ½ cup avocado oil
- ❖ 1 egg, whisked

- ❖ Salt and black pepper to the taste
- ❖ 1 cup asiago cheese, shredded
- ❖ ¼ teaspoon garlic powder
- ❖ 1 cup parmesan cheese, grated

INSTRUCTIONS

1. In a bowl, mix parmesan cheese with garlic, salt and pepper and stir.
2. Put whisked egg in another bowl and mix with the water.
3. Season chicken with salt and pepper and dip each piece into egg and then into cheese mix.
4. Heat up a pan with the oil over medium high heat, add chicken breasts, cook until they are golden on both sides and transfer to a baking pan.
5. Introduce in the oven at 350 degrees F and bake for 20 minutes.
6. Top chicken with bacon and asiago cheese, introduce in the oven, turn on broiler and broil for a couple of minutes.
7. Serve hot.

Brussels sprouts and hamburger gratin

Made for: Dinner | Prep Time: 55 minutes | Servings: 4 people
Nutrition Per Servings: Kcal: 766, Protein: 45g, Fat: 63g, Net Carb: 7g

INGREDIENTS

- ❖ 1 lb ground beef
- ❖ ½ lb bacon, diced
- ❖ 1 lb Brussels sprouts, cut in halves
- ❖ 4 tbsp sour cream
- ❖ 2 oz. butter
- ❖ 5 oz. shredded cheese
- ❖ 1 tbsp Italian seasoning
- ❖ salt and pepper

INSTRUCTIONS

1. Set the oven to 425°F (220°C).
2. Fry the bacon and Brussels sprouts in butter. Season and stir in sour cream. Place in a baking dish.
3. Fry the ground beef golden-brown, season with salt and pepper and sprinkle on top of the Brussels sprouts. Add cheese and herbs.
4. Place in the middle of the oven for 15 minutes or until done. Serve with a fresh salad and maybe a dollop of mayonnaise.

Delicious Chicken Wings

Made for: Dinner | Prep Time: 65 minutes | Servings: 4 people
Nutrition Per Servings: Kcal: 415, Protein: 28g, Fat: 23g, Net Carb: 2g

INGREDIENTS

- ❖ 3 pounds chicken wings
- ❖ Salt and black pepper to the taste
- ❖ 3 tablespoons coconut aminos
- ❖ 2 teaspoons white vinegar
- ❖ 3 tablespoons rice vinegar
- ❖ 3 tablespoons stevia
- ❖ ¼ cup scallions, chopped
- ❖ ½ teaspoon xanthan gum 5 dried chilies, chopped

INSTRUCTIONS

1. Spread chicken wings on a lined baking sheet, season with salt and pepper, introduce in the oven at 375 degrees F and bake for 45 minutes.
2. Meanwhile, heat up a small pan over medium heat, add white vinegar, rice vinegar, coconut aminos, stevia, xanthan gum, scallions and chilies, stir well, bring to a boil, cook for 2 minutes and take off heat.
3. Dip chicken wings into this sauce, arrange them all on the baking sheet again and bake for 10 minutes more.
4. Serve them hot.

Keto zucchini pizza boats

Made for: Dinner | Prep Time: 35 minutes | Servings: 2 people
Nutrition Per Servings: Kcal: 692, Protein: 29g, Fat: 61g, Net Carb: 4g

INGREDIENTS

- ❖ 1 medium-sized zucchini
- ❖ 2 garlic cloves, sliced thinly
- ❖ 4 tbsp olive oil
- ❖ 1½ oz. baby spinach
- ❖ salt and pepper to taste
- ❖ 2 tbsp unsweetened marinara sauce
- ❖ 8 oz. goat cheese

INSTRUCTIONS

1. Preheat oven to 375°F (190°C).
2. Slice the zucchini in half, length-wise, and use a spoon to scrape out the seeds (don't throw them away!). Put the zucchini boats on a baking sheet.
3. Fry the garlic in a skillet, with about half of the olive oil over medium heat, until lightly browned. Add the baby spinach and zucchini seeds. Fry until soft. Season with a pinch of salt and ground black pepper.
4. Spread the marinara sauce over the zucchini boats, and top with the fried baby spinach and garlic. Sprinkle the goat cheese on top.
5. Bake for about 20–25 minutes or until the zucchini is as tender as you'd prefer and the cheese has a nice golden color.
6. Drizzle the zucchini boats with the rest of the olive oil and season with some freshly ground black pepper before serving.

Keto pizza chaffles

Made for: Dinner | Prep Time: 25 minutes | Servings: 4 people
Nutrition Per Servings: Kcal: 430, Protein: 29g, Fat: 31g, Net Carb: 2g

INGREDIENTS

Pizza chaffles
- ❖ 4 eggs
- ❖ 8 oz. (1 cup equals 4 oz) cheddar cheese, shredded

- ❖ ½ tsp Italian seasoning
- ❖ 1 oz. parmesan cheese, grated

Topping
- ❖ 4 tsp tomato sauce, sugar free
- ❖ 16 pepperoni slices

- ❖ 3 oz. mozzarella cheese, shredded

INSTRUCTIONS

1. Pre-heat your waffle maker.
2. Place all of your ingredients into a mixing bowl and beat to combine well.
3. Lightly grease your waffle iron and then evenly spoon the mixture over the bottom plate, spreading it out slightly to get an even result. Close the waffle iron and cook for approx 6 minutes, depending on your waffle maker.
4. Gently lift the lid when you think they're done.
5. Line a large baking tray with parchment paper and place the chaffles on it.
6. Spread each chaffle with tomato sauce and top with pepperoni slices and mozzarella.
7. Place under a hot grill until the cheese is browned and bubbly (approx. 2 minutes).

Fried chicken with broccoli

Made for: Dinner | Prep Time: 25 minutes | Servings: 4 people
Nutrition Per Servings: Kcal: 732, Protein: 30g, Fat: 66g, Net Carb: 5g

INGREDIENTS

- ❖ 9 oz. broccoli
- ❖ 3½ oz. butter
- ❖ 10 oz. boneless chicken thighs
- ❖ salt and pepper
- ❖ ½ cup mayonnaise, for serving (optional)

INSTRUCTIONS

1. Rinse and trim the broccoli. Cut into smaller pieces, including the stem.
2. Heat up a generous dollop of butter in a frying pan where you can fit both the chicken and the broccoli.
3. Season the chicken and fry over medium heat for about 5 minutes per side, or until golden brown and cooked through.
4. Add more butter and put the broccoli in the same frying pan. Fry for another couple of minutes.
5. Season to taste and serve with the remaining butter.

Fried salmon with broccoli

Made for: Dinner | Prep Time: 5 minutes | Servings: 4 people
Nutrition Per Servings: Kcal: 685, Protein: 41g, Fat: 53g, Net Carb: 5g

INGREDIENTS

- ❖ 1 lb broccoli
- ❖ 3 oz. butter
- ❖ salt and pepper
- ❖ 5 oz. grated cheddar cheese
- ❖ 1½ lbs salmon
- ❖ 1 lime (optional)

INSTRUCTIONS

1. Preheat the oven to 400°F (200°C), preferably using the broiler setting.

2. Cut the broccoli into smaller florets and let simmer in lightly salted water for a couple of minutes. Make sure the broccoli maintains its chewy texture and delicate color.

3. Drain the broccoli and discard the boiling water. Set aside, uncovered, for a minute or two to allow the steam to evaporate.

4. Place the drained broccoli in a well-greased baking dish. Add butter and pepper to taste.

5. Sprinkle cheese on top of the broccoli and bake in the oven for 15-20 minutes or until the cheese turns a golden color.

6. In the meantime, season the salmon with salt and pepper and fry in plenty of butter, a few minutes on each side. The lime can be fried in the same pan or be served raw. This step can also be made on an outdoor grill.

Chicken with lemon and butter

Made for: Dinner | Prep Time: 60 minutes | Servings: 4 people
Nutrition Per Servings: Kcal: 998, Protein: 62g, Fat: 81g, Net Carb: 0.5g

INGREDIENTS

- ❖ 3 lbs chicken whole
- ❖ salt and pepper
- ❖ 2 tsp barbecue seasoning dry rub
- ❖ 5 oz. butter sliced
- ❖ 1 lemon, cut into wedges
- ❖ 2 yellow onions cut into wedges
- ❖ ¼ cup water
- ❖ 1 tsp butter for greasing the baking dish

INSTRUCTIONS

1. Preheat the oven to 350°F (175°C). Grease a deep baking dish with butter.

2. Prepare the chicken by drying it thoroughly with paper towels. Season the entire chicken with salt and pepper, including the cavity. Don't skimp on the salt! Next rub the outside of the chicken with the barbecue seasoning, and then place it in the baking dish.

3. Surround the chicken with the onion and lemon wedges, and then evenly place the butter slices on top of the chicken.

4. Move the baking dish to the lower oven rack, and bake for 1½ hours or more, depending on the size of the chicken. Frequently baste the chicken with drippings, and if necessary, add water. If testing the chicken for readiness with a kitchen thermometer, insert it into the thickest part of the thigh, avoiding the bone. The chicken is ready when the temperature reads 165°F (75°C).

Grilled Squid and Tasty Guacamole

Made for: Dinner | Prep Time: 25 minutes | Servings: 2 people
Nutrition Per Servings: Kcal: 510, Protein: 25g, Fat: 44g, Net Carb: 6g

INGREDIENTS

- ❖ 2 medium squids, tentacles separated and tubes scored lengthwise
- ❖ A drizzle of olive oil
- ❖ Juice from 1 lime
- ❖ Salt and black pepper to the taste
- ❖ For the guacamole:
- ❖ 2 avocados, pitted, peeled and chopped
- ❖ Some coriander springs, chopped
- ❖ 2 red chilies, chopped
- ❖ 1 tomato, chopped
- ❖ 1 red onion, chopped Juice from 2 limes

INSTRUCTIONS

1. Season squid and squid tentacles with salt, pepper, drizzle some olive oil and massage well.
2. Place on preheated grill over medium high heat score side down and cook for 2 minutes.
3. Flip and cook for 2 minutes more and transfer to a bowl.
4. Add juice from 1 lime, toss to coat and keep warm.
5. Put avocado in a bowl and mash using a fork.
6. Add coriander, chilies, tomato, onion and juice from 2 limes and stir well everything.
7. Divide squid on plates, top with guacamole and serve.

Spicy keto chicken casserole

Made for: Dinner | Prep Time: 40 minutes | Servings: 2 people
Nutrition Per Servings: Kcal: 1139, Protein: 78g, Fat: 82g, Net Carb: 10g

INGREDIENTS

- ❖ 1 lb chicken breasts (without skin), cut into bite-sized pieces
- ❖ 5 oz. bacon, coarsely chopped
- ❖ 1 garlic clove, pressed
- ❖ 2 oz. broccoli, cut into small florets
- ❖ 3 oz. cauliflower, cut into small florets
- ❖ 1 tsp sambal oelek
- ❖ 1 tbsp tomato paste
- ❖ 1 cup heavy whipping cream
- ❖ 2 oz. shredded cheese
- ❖ salt and pepper
- ❖ butter, to grease casserole dish

For serving

- ❖ 2 oz. leafy greens
- ❖ ½ small red onion, divided and thinly sliced
- ❖ 3 oz. cherry tomatoes, cut into quarts

INSTRUCTIONS

1. Preheat the oven to 400°F (200°C). Lightly grease a 9 x 12 casserole dish with butter.
2. Heat a large frying pan over medium heat. Add the bacon and fry until crispy. Remove from pan and distribute it in a casserole dish.
3. Using the bacon fat, fry the chicken together with garlic and salt and pepper for about 15 minutes, until chicken is no longer pink. Add chicken to the casserole dish.
4. Distribute cauliflower and broccoli evenly among the chicken in the baking dish.
5. In a saucepan over medium heat, whisk together heavy whipping cream, tomato paste, and sambal oelek. Season with salt and pepper and bring to a boil.
6. Pour the sauce into the baking dish, distributing well among chicken, vegetables, and bacon.
7. Cover with foil to prevent from burning. Bake in the oven for 30 minutes.
8. Remove the aluminum foil and add shredded cheese on the top of the casserole. Put the baking dish back into the oven, uncovered, and bake for about 15 minutes or until the cheese is bubbly and light gold.
9. Serve with a fresh salad.

Scrambled eggs with basil and butter

Made for: Dinner | Prep Time: 15 minutes | Servings: 2 people
Nutrition Per Servings: Kcal: 642, Protein: 24g, Fat: 60g, Net Carb: 2g

INGREDIENTS

- ❖ 4 tbsp butter
- ❖ 4 eggs
- ❖ 4 tbsp heavy whipping cream
- ❖ salt and ground black pepper
- ❖ 4 oz. shredded cheese
- ❖ 4 tbsp fresh basil

INSTRUCTIONS

1. Melt butter in a pan on low heat.
2. Add cracked eggs, cream, shredded cheese, and seasoning to a small bowl. Give it a light whisk and add to the pan.

3. Stir with a spatula from the edge towards the center until the eggs are scrambled. If you prefer it soft and creamy, stir on lower heat until desired consistency.

4. Top with fresh basil.

Keto Croque Monsieur

Made for: Dinner | Prep Time: 25 minutes | Servings: 2 people
Nutrition Per Servings: Kcal: 1089, Protein: 50g, Fat: 90g, Net Carb: 8g

INGREDIENTS

- ❖ 8 oz. cottage cheese
- ❖ 4 eggs
- ❖ 1 tbsp ground psyllium husk powder
- ❖ 4 tbsp butter or coconut oil for frying
- ❖ 5⅓ oz. smoked deli ham
- ❖ 5⅓ oz. cheddar cheese
- ❖ ½ finely chopped red onion (optional)

INSTRUCTIONS

1. Whisk the eggs in a bowl. Mix in the cottage cheese. Add ground psyllium husk powder while stirring to incorporate it smoothly, without lumps. Let the mixture rest for five minutes until the batter has set.

2. Place a frying pan over medium heat. Add a generous amount of butter and fry the batter like small pancakes for a couple of minutes on each side, until they are golden. Make two pancakes per serving.

3. Assemble a sandwich with sliced ham and cheese between two of the warm pancakes. Add finely chopped onion on top.

4. Wash and tear the lettuce. Mix oil, vinegar, salt and pepper into a simple vinaigrette. Serve the Croque Monsieur warm beside lettuce dressed with the vinaigrette.

Fried eggs with kale

Made for: Dinner | Prep Time: 40 minutes | Servings: 2 people
Nutrition Per Servings: Kcal: 1032, Protein: 25g, Fat: 98g, Net Carb: 6g

INGREDIENTS

- ❖ ½ lb kale
- ❖ 3 oz. butter
- ❖ 6 oz. smoked pork belly or bacon

- ❖ 1 oz. frozen cranberries
- ❖ 1 oz. pecans or walnuts
- ❖ 4 eggs
- ❖ salt and pepper

INSTRUCTIONS

1. Trim and chop the kale into large squares. (Pre-washed baby kale is a terrific shortcut.) Melt two thirds of the butter in a frying pan and fry the kale quickly on high heat until slightly browned around the edges.
2. Remove the kale from the frying pan and set aside. Sear the pork belly or bacon in the same frying pan until crispy.
3. Lower the heat. Return the sautéed kale to the pan and add the cranberries and nuts. Stir until warmed through. Reserve in a bowl.
4. Turn up the heat and fry the eggs in the rest of the butter. Salt and pepper to taste. Plate two fried eggs with each portion of greens and serve immediately

Snacks & Desserts Recipes

Keto hot chocolate

Prep Time: 10 minutes | Servings: 01 people
Nutrition Per Servings: Kcal: 219, Protein: 2g, Fat: 21g, Net Carb: 1g

INGREDIENTS

- ❖ 1 oz. unsalted butter
- ❖ 1 tbsp cocoa powder
- ❖ 2½ tsp powdered erythritol
- ❖ ¼ tsp vanilla extract

- ❖ 1 cup boiling water

INSTRUCTIONS

1. Put the ingredients in a tall beaker to use with an immersion blender.
2. Mix for 15–20 seconds or until there's a fine foam on top.
3. Pour the hot cocoa carefully into to cups and enjoy.

Carrot Cake Keto Balls

Prep Time: 20 minutes | Servings: 16 people
Nutrition Per Servings: Kcal: 132, Protein: 5g, Fat: 12g, Net Carb: 1g

INGREDIENTS

- ❖ 1 (8-oz.) block cream cheese, softened
- ❖ 3/4 c. coconut flour
- ❖ 1 tsp. stevia
- ❖ 1/2 tsp. pure vanilla extract
- ❖ 1 tsp. cinnamon
- ❖ 1/4 tsp. ground nutmeg
- ❖ 1 c. grated carrots
- ❖ 1/2 c. chopped pecans
- ❖ 1 c. shredded unsweetened coconut

INSTRUCTIONS

1. In a large bowl, using a hand mixer, beat together cream cheese, coconut flour, stevia, vanilla, cinnamon, and nutmeg. Fold in carrots and pecans.
2. Roll into 16 balls then roll in shredded coconut and serve.

Keto cinnamon coffee

Prep Time: 10 minutes | Servings: 02 people
Nutrition Per Servings: Kcal: 135, Protein: 2g, Fat: 12g, Net Carb: 1g

INGREDIENTS

- ❖ 2 tbsp ground coffee
- ❖ 1 tsp ground cinnamon
- ❖ 2 cups water
- ❖ 1/3 cup heavy whipping cream

INSTRUCTIONS

1. Mix ground coffee and cinnamon. Add piping hot water and brew as usual.
2. Whip the cream using a whisk or a mixer until medium stiff peaks form.
3. Serve the coffee in a tall mug (a glass mug is fun if you have it) and add the whipped cream on top. Finish with a small sprinkle of ground cinnamon.

Keto Tortilla Chips

Prep Time: 35 minutes | Servings: 04 people
Nutrition Per Servings: Kcal: 623, Protein: 21g, Fat: 54g, Net Carb: 4g

INGREDIENTS

- ❖ 2 c. shredded mozzarella
- ❖ 1 c. almond flour
- ❖ 1 tsp. kosher salt
- ❖ 1 tsp. garlic powder
- ❖ 1/2 tsp. chili powder
- ❖ Freshly ground black pepper

INSTRUCTIONS

1. Preheat oven to 350°. Line two large baking sheets with parchment paper.
2. In a microwave safe bowl, melt mozzarella, about 1 minute 30 seconds. Add almond flour, salt, garlic powder, chili powder, and a few cracks black pepper. Using your hands, knead dough a few times until a smooth ball forms.
3. Place dough between two sheets of parchment paper and roll out into a rectangle ⅛" thick. Using a knife or pizza cutter, cut dough into triangles.
4. Spread chips out on prepared baking sheets and bake until edges are golden and starting to crisp, 12 to 14 minutes.

Avocado Chips

Prep Time: 45 minutes | Servings: 15 people

Nutrition Per Servings: 120 calories, 7 g protein, 4 g carbohydrates, 2 g fiber, 0 g sugar, 10 g fat

INGREDIENTS

- ❖ 1 large ripe avocado
- ❖ 3/4 c. freshly grated Parmesan
- ❖ 1 tsp. lemon juice
- ❖ 1/2 tsp. garlic powder
- ❖ 1/2 tsp. Italian seasoning
- ❖ Kosher salt
- ❖ Freshly ground black pepper

INSTRUCTIONS

1. Preheat oven to 325° and line two baking sheets with parchment paper. In a medium bowl, mash avocado with a fork until smooth. Stir in Parmesan, lemon juice, garlic powder, and Italian seasoning. Season with salt and pepper.
2. Place heaping teaspoon-size scoops of mixture on baking sheet, leaving about 3" apart between each scoop. Flatten each scoop to 3" wide across with the back of a spoon or measuring cup. Bake until crisp and golden, about 30 minutes, then let cool completely. Serve at room temperature.

Keto Smoothie

Prep Time: 15 minutes | Servings: 04 people

Nutrition Per Servings: Kcal: 175, Protein: 5g, Fat: 7g, Net Carb: 1g

INGREDIENTS

- 1 1/2 c. frozen strawberries
- 1 1/2 c. frozen raspberries, plus more for garnish (optional)
- 1 c. frozen blackberries
- 2 c. coconut milk
- 1 c. baby spinach
- Unsweetened shaved coconut, for garnish (optional)

INSTRUCTIONS

1. In a blender, combine all ingredients (except for coconut). Blend until smooth.
2. Divide between cups and top with raspberries and coconut, if using.

Keto spinach dip

Prep Time: 10 minutes | Servings: 06 people
Nutrition Per Servings: Kcal: 312, Protein: 1g, Fat: 34g, Net Carb: 2g

INGREDIENTS

- ❖ 2 tbsp light olive oil
- ❖ 2 oz. frozen spinach
- ❖ 2 tbsp dried parsley
- ❖ 1 tbsp dried dill
- ❖ 1 tsp onion powder
- ❖ ½ tsp salt
- ❖ ¼ tsp ground black pepper
- ❖ 1 cup mayonnaise
- ❖ ¼ cup sour cream
- ❖ 2 tsp lemon juice

INSTRUCTIONS

1. Thaw the frozen spinach and remove excessive liquid.
2. Place in a bowl and mix with the other ingredients.
3. Let sit for 10 minutes to let the flavors develop.

Spicy keto roasted nuts

Prep Time: 15 minutes | Servings: 06 people
Nutrition Per Servings: Kcal: 285, Protein: 4g, Fat: 30g, Net Carb: 2g

INGREDIENTS

- ❖ 8 oz. pecans or almonds or walnuts
- ❖ 1 tsp salt

- ❖ 1 tbsp olive oil or coconut oil
- ❖ 1 tsp ground cumin
- ❖ 1 tsp paprika powder or chili powder

INSTRUCTIONS

1. Mix all ingredients in a medium frying pan, and cook on medium heat until the almonds are warmed through.
2. Let cool and serve as a snack with a drink. Store in a container with lid at room temperature.

Keto bread twists

Prep Time: 40 minutes | Servings: 10 people
Nutrition Per Servings: Kcal: 195, Protein: 7g, Fat: 17g, Net Carb: 1g

INGREDIENTS

- ❖ ½ cup almond flour
- ❖ ¼ cup coconut flour
- ❖ ½ tsp salt
- ❖ 1 tsp baking powder
- ❖ 1 egg, beaten
- ❖ 2 oz. butter
- ❖ 6½ oz. shredded cheese, preferably mozzarella
- ❖ ¼ cup green pesto
- ❖ 1 egg, beaten, for brushing the top

INSTRUCTIONS

1. Preheat the oven to 350°F (175°C).
2. Mix all dry ingredients in a bowl. Add the egg and combine.
3. Melt the butter and the cheese together in a pot on low heat. Stir until the batter is smooth.
4. Slowly add the butter-cheese batter to the dry mixture bowl and mix together into a firm dough.
5. Place the dough on parchment paper that is the size of a rectangular cookie sheet. Use a rolling pin and make a rectangle, about 1/5-inch (5 mm) thick.
6. Spread pesto on top and cut into 1-inch (2.5 cm) strips. Twist them and place on a baking sheet lined with parchment paper. Brush twists with the whisked egg.
7. Bake in the oven for 15–20 minutes until they're golden brown.

Keto cheese chips

Prep Time: 15 minutes | Servings: 04 people
Nutrition Per Servings: Kcal: 231, Protein: 13g, Fat: 19g, Net Carb: 2g

INGREDIENTS

- ❖ 8 oz. cheddar cheese or provolone cheese or edam cheese, shredded
- ❖ ½ tsp paprika powder

INSTRUCTIONS

1. Preheat the oven to 400°F (200°C).
2. Add shredded cheese in small heaps on a baking sheet lined with parchment paper. Make sure to leave enough room in between them so they aren't touching.
3. Sprinkle paprika powder on top and bake in the oven for about 8–10 minutes, depending on how thick they are. Pay attention towards the end so that you don't burn the cheese, as burned cheese tends to have a bitter taste.
4. Let cool on a cooling rack, and enjoy — great alone as a crunchy snack or perfect to serve with a dip.

Keto avocado hummus

Prep Time: 10 minutes | Servings: 06 people
Nutrition Per Servings: Kcal: 417, Protein: 05g, Fat: 41g, Net Carb: 4g

INGREDIENTS

- ❖ 3 ripe avocados
- ❖ ½ cup fresh cilantro
- ❖ ½ cup olive oil
- ❖ ¼ cup sunflower seeds
- ❖ ¼ cup tahini (sesame paste)
- ❖ 1 tbsp lemon juice
- ❖ 1 garlic clove, pressed
- ❖ ½ tsp ground cumin
- ❖ ½ tsp salt
- ❖ ¼ tsp ground black pepper

1. Cut the avocado lengthwise, remove the pit and spoon out the flesh.
2. Put all ingredients in a blender or food processor and mix until thoroughly smooth.
3. Add more oil, lemon juice or water if you want to have a looser texture. Adjust seasonings as needed.

Vegan & Vegetarian Recipes

Roasted cabbage

Prep Time: 40 minutes | Servings: 04 people
Nutrition Per Servings: Kcal: 367, Protein: 3g, Fat: 62g, Net Carb: 7g

INGREDIENTS

- ❖ 2 lbs green cabbage
- ❖ 6 oz. butter
- ❖ 1 tsp salt
- ❖ ¼ tsp ground black pepper

INSTRUCTIONS

1. Preheat the oven to 400°F (200°C).
2. Melt the butter in a sauce pan over medium-low heat.
3. Split the green cabbage into wedges and remove the thick stem in the middle. Cut slices — less than an inch thick — and place on a baking sheet lined with parchment paper or in a large baking dish.
4. Season with salt and pepper and pour the melted butter on top.
5. Bake for 20 minutes or until the cabbage is roasted.

Spicy keto deviled eggs

Prep Time: 30 minutes | Servings: 06 people
Nutrition Per Servings: Kcal: 210, Protein: 6g, Fat: 19g, Net Carb: 1g

INGREDIENTS

- ❖ 6 eggs
- ❖ 1 tbsp red curry paste
- ❖ ½ cup mayonnaise
- ❖ ¼ tsp salt

❖ ½ tbsp poppy seeds

INSTRUCTIONS

1. Place the eggs in cold water in a pan, just enough water to cover the eggs. Bring to a boil without a lid.
2. Let the eggs simmer for about eight minutes. Cool quickly in ice-cold water.
3. Remove the egg shells. Cut off both ends and split the egg in half. Scoop out the egg yolk and place in a small bowl.
4. Place the egg whites on a plate and let sit in the refrigerator.
5. Mix curry paste, mayonnaise and egg yolks into a smooth batter. Salt to taste.
6. Bring out the egg whites from the refrigerator and apply the batter.
7. Sprinkle the seeds on top and serve.

Cauliflower Hash Browns

Prep Time: 35 minutes | Servings: 09 people
Nutrition Per Servings: Kcal: 101, Protein: 3g, Fat: 6g, Net Carb: 5g

INGREDIENTS

❖ 1 head cauliflower, riced (about 3 cups) – See Notes
❖ 2 tablespoons almond flour
❖ 1 tablespoon coconut flour
❖ 3 organic eggs
❖ 1/2 teaspoon garlic powder
❖ 1 teaspoon fine sea salt
❖ 1/2 teaspoon black pepper
❖ Avocado oil, for frying

INSTRUCTIONS

1. In a food processor, or using a hand grater, pulse/grate cauliflower until rice consistency.
2. In a bowl combine eggs, cauliflower rice, almond flour, coconut flour, garlic powder, and salt and pepper.
3. Heat skillet over medium heat. Once hot add oil to coat pan.
4. Scoop 1/4 cup of cauliflower mixture and form into hashbrown shaped patties approximately 3/4-inch thick and gently place in skillet. Repeat with remaining mixture, cooking in batches as necessary.

5. Cook hash browns until golden brown, approximately 3-4 minutes per side.
6. Serve immediately or cool and freeze for future use.

Roasted Vegetable Scramble

Prep Time: 50 minutes | Servings: 02 people
Nutrition Per Servings: Kcal: 256, Protein: 5g, Fat: 11g, Net Carb: 1g

INGREDIENTS

- ❖ 1 tablespoon avocado oil or olive oil
- ❖ 1 medium zucchini squash halved lengthwise and chopped
- ❖ 1 medium yellow squash halved lengthwise and chopped
- ❖ 2 carrots peeled and chopped

- ❖ 4 cups baby spinach loosely packed
- ❖ 6 large eggs well beaten.
- ❖ sea salt to taste
- ❖ 1/2 ripe avocado sliced

INSTRUCTIONS

1. Preheat the oven to 420 degrees F. Place chopped zucchini squash, yellow squash, and carrots on a large baking sheet and drizzle with avocado oil and sprinkle with sea salt. Use your hands to toss everything together until the vegetables are well coated. Spread vegetables into a single layer on the baking sheet. Roast 20 to 25 minutes in the preheated oven, until golden brown. Remove from oven.
2. Heat a medium-sized skillet over medium heat with enough oil to lightly coat the surface, about 2 teaspoons. Add the baby spinach and cover. Cook, stirring occasionally, until wilted, about 2 minutes. Transfer the roasted vegetables to the skillet. Evenly pour the beaten eggs over the vegetables and sprinkle liberally with sea salt. Allow eggs to sit untouched for 1 to 2 minutes. Use a spatula to flip the eggs and cook another 1 to 2 minutes. Continue cooking and flipping until eggs are cooked through.
3. Serve scramble with fresh fruit and sliced avocado

Warm keto kale salad

Prep Time: 30 minutes | Servings: 04 people
Nutrition Per Servings: Kcal: 488, Protein: 10g, Fat: 48g, Net Carb: 5g

INGREDIENTS

- ❖ ¾ cup heavy whipping cream
- ❖ 2 tbsp mayonnaise
- ❖ 1 tsp Dijon mustard

- ❖ 2 tbsp olive oil
- ❖ 1 garlic clove, minced or finely chopped
- ❖ salt and pepper

- ❖ 2 oz. butter
- ❖ 8 oz. kale
- ❖ 4 oz. blue cheese or feta cheese

INSTRUCTIONS

1. Mix together heavy cream, mayonnaise, mustard, olive oil and garlic in a small beaker. Salt and pepper to taste.
2. Rinse the kale and cut into small, bite-size pieces. Remove and discard the thick stem.
3. Heat a large frying pan and add the butter. Sauté the kale quickly so it turns a nice color, but no more than that. Salt and pepper to taste.
4. Place in a bowl and pour the dressing on top. Stir thoroughly and serve with crumbled blue cheese or another flavorful cheese of your choice.

Broccoli Cheese Bites

Prep Time: 50 minutes | Servings: 24 people
Nutrition Per Servings: Kcal: 49, Protein: 4g, Fat: 5g, Net Carb: 1g

INGREDIENTS

- ❖ 2 heads Broccoli
- ❖ 1/2 cup frozen spinach defrosted and drained well
- ❖ 1/4 cup Scallions sliced
- ❖ 1 Lemon Zest only
- ❖ 1 cup Cheddar Cheese grated

- ❖ 1/4 cup Parmesan cheese grated
- ❖ 2 eggs
- ❖ 1/3 cup Sour Cream
- ❖ 1/2 teaspoon Pepper
- ❖ 1/4 teaspoon Salt

INSTRUCTIONS

1. Preheat oven to 180C/355F.
2. Cut broccoli into evenly sized florets and place in a microwave safe container with ¼ cup of water. Microwave on high for 3 minutes or until the broccoli is tender. Drain well and allow to cool.
3. Chop the broccoli into very small pieces, You should end up with approximately 2-2 ½ cups.
4. Place the chopped broccoli in a bowl with all the remaining ingredients and mix well.
5. Pour the mixture into a 11 x 7in rectangle brownie pan, lined with parchment paper, and smooth into an even layer.
6. Bake for 25 minutes, until the bites are puffed and browning.
7. Allow to cool for 10 minutes, before cutting into 24 squares.

Keto Broccoli & Leek Soup Recipe

Prep Time: 20 minutes | Servings: 05 people
Nutrition Per Servings: Kcal: 268, Protein: 8g, Fat: 24g, Net Carb: 6g

INGREDIENTS

- ❖ 1 medium Leek white part only
- ❖ 1 clove garlic
- ❖ 3 ounces Butter salted
- ❖ 1 pound Broccoli 2 medium heads
- ❖ 1/2 cup Heavy Cream

- ❖ 2 1/2 cups chicken stock
- ❖ 1 tsp Salt
- ❖ 1 tsp Pepper
- ❖ 1 tbsp Parsley chopped

INSTRUCTIONS

1. Roughly chop the white part of the leek and place into a large saucepan, along with the butter and garlic.
2. Saute the leeks over low heat until they are beginning to turn translucent. Add the cream.
3. Cut the broccoli into evenly sized florets and place into the saucepan.
4. Add the chicken stock and stir. Ensure that the broccoli is mostly covered.
5. Simmer on low to medium heat for 8 minutes. If you cook the broccoli too quick, it will discolor and turn the soup an off brown color. The broccoli is cooked when it is easy to break up with a spoon.
6. Using a stick blender, carefully blend the soup until no lumps are remaining.
7. Stir through the salt, pepper, and parsley. Adjust seasoning to taste. Enjoy.

Buttery Bacon and Cabbage Stir Fry

Prep Time: 20 minutes | Servings: 01 people
Nutrition Per Servings: Kcal: 378, Protein: 3g, Fat: 41g, Net Carb: 3g

INGREDIENTS

- ❖ 50 g Butter
- ❖ 150 g Napa Cabbage shredded
- ❖ 2 rashers bacon

- ❖ 1 pinch Salt
- ❖ 1 pinch Pepper

INSTRUCTIONS

1. Dice bacon and add to frying pan on medium heat, along with half of butter. Saute bacon until crisp.
2. Add shredded cabbage to bacon and stir well to ensure the cabbage is coated in the pan juices.

3. Add the other half of butter to pan along with a pinch of pepper and cook until cabbage is becoming translucent.
4. Taste to adjust seasonings and serve. You may not wish to add any salt, depending on the saltiness of the bacon used.

Broccoli Mash

Prep Time: 20 minutes | Servings: 04 people
Nutrition Per Servings: Kcal: 134, Protein: 4g, Fat: 10g, Net Carb: 9g

INGREDIENTS

- ❖ 1 pound Broccoli 2 medium heads
- ❖ 1/2 teaspoon Salt
- ❖ 1/2 teaspoon Pepper
- ❖ 1 ounce Butter
- ❖ 3 ounces Sour Cream
- ❖ 2 tablespoons chives finely chopped

INSTRUCTIONS

1. Bring a large pot of water to the boil.
2. Cut the broccoli into evenly sized florets.
3. Gently add the broccoli to the boiling water and cook for 3-5 minutes, until the broccoli is tender.
4. Drain the broccoli and return it to the warm pot, add the butter, sour cream, salt and pepper.
5. Blend the broccoli with a stick blender until there are no lumps.
6. Stir through the chives and adjust the seasoning.

Keto Vegetable Soup

Prep Time: 45 minutes | Servings: 10 people
Nutrition Per Servings: Kcal: 75, Protein: 4g, Fat: 3g, Net Carb: 5g

INGREDIENTS

- ❖ 1 tablespoon butter
- ❖ 1 tablespoon olive oil
- ❖ 1 medium onion, chopped
- ❖ 3 stalks celery, chopped
- ❖ 2 carrots, peeled and chopped
- ❖ 4 cloves garlic, minced
- ❖ 2 cups chopped cauliflower florets
- ❖ 1 ½ cups fresh green beans, trimmed and cut into 1 inch pieces
- ❖ 30 ounces canned diced tomatoes
- ❖ 8 cups beef broth
- ❖ 1 tablespoon Worcestershire sauce
- ❖ 1 tablespoon Italian seasoning
- ❖ 1 teaspoon salt
- ❖ 1 teaspoon cracked pepper
- ❖ 2 cups fresh spinach

INSTRUCTIONS

1. Add the butter and olive to a large stock pot over medium heat until butter has melted.
2. Add the onions, celery, carrots, and garlic and cook for 5 minutes, stirring often.
3. Add the cauliflower, green beans, tomatoes, beef broth, Worcestershire sauce, and Italian seasoning. Stir to combine.
4. Bring to a boil, reduce to a simmer, and cook for 25 minutes or until vegetable are tender.
5. Season with the salt and pepper and add the spinach to the pot. Stir well and continue cooking for 1-2 minutes until the spinach has wilted.
6. Taste and add additional salt and pepper, if needed. Serve immediately.

Low Carb Broccoli and Bacon Croquettes

Prep Time: 14 minutes | Servings: 60 people
Nutrition Per Servings: Kcal: 126, Protein: 8g, Fat: 10g, Net Carb: 3g

INGREDIENTS

- ❖ 1 lb Broccoli
- ❖ 2 oz Butter
- ❖ 3 slices bacon
- ❖ 1/2 cup parmesan grated
- ❖ 1 Egg

- ❖ 2 oz Pork Rinds crushed into crumbs
- ❖ 1 tsp Salt
- ❖ 2 tsp Pepper
- ❖ 1 tbsp Flaxseed ground
- ❖ 1 tbsp almond meal

INSTRUCTIONS

1. Boil or steam broccoli for 5 minutes, or until tender, Drain well.
2. Blend the warm broccoli with the butter into a puree. Place into a bowl and stir through the grated parmesan, pepper and salt.
3. Dice the bacon into small pieces and saute over a low to medium heat for 6 to 8 minutes. The bacon fat will render whilst the bacon browns, add the bacon and fat to the broccoli and mix well.
4. Chill the broccoli and bacon mix for at least 30 minutes.
5. Turn your deep fryer to 350F/180C and allow to heat up.
6. After the mix has chilled, add the egg and ground up pork rinds and mix well.
7. Roll the mixture into 14 small barrel shapes.
8. On a plate mix together the almond meal and flaxseed meal, roll each croquette through this dry mix and ensure each side is coated, pressing the mixture onto the surface of the croquette.
9. Deep fry your croquettes in batches, ensuring you don't overcrowd the fryer. They will take around 3-5 minutes, remove when crisp and golden brown. Enjoy!

Broccoli Cheese Bites

Prep Time: 40 minutes | Servings: 24 people

Nutrition Per Servings: Kcal: 59, Protein: 4g, Fat: 5g, Net Carb: 1g

INGREDIENTS

- ❖ 2 heads Broccoli
- ❖ 1/2 cup frozen spinach defrosted and drained well
- ❖ 1/4 cup Scallions sliced
- ❖ 1 Lemon Zest only
- ❖ 1 cup Cheddar Cheese grated

- ❖ 1/4 cup Parmesan cheese grated
- ❖ 2 eggs
- ❖ 1/3 cup Sour Cream
- ❖ 1/2 teaspoon Pepper
- ❖ 1/4 teaspoon Salt

INSTRUCTIONS

1. Preheat oven to 180C/355F.
2. Cut broccoli into evenly sized florets and place in a microwave safe container with ¼ cup of water. Microwave on high for 3 minutes or until the broccoli is tender. Drain well and allow to cool.
3. Chop the broccoli into very small pieces, You should end up with approximately 2-2 ½ cups.
4. Place the chopped broccoli in a bowl with all the remaining ingredients and mix well.
5. Pour the mixture into a 11 x 7in rectangle brownie pan, lined with parchment paper, and smooth into an even layer.
6. Bake for 25 minutes, until the bites are puffed and browning.
7. Allow to cool for 10 minutes, before cutting into 24 squares.

CONCLUSION

One of the primary keys to any successful diet or lifestyle change has always been the recipes that fit in with the principles of the diet. I am sure there are many ways to achieve ketosis and to attain that weight loss goal. However, you do not want to get there by just having the same old dishes over and over again.

Variety is the name of the game here, which is crucial in ensuring the sustainability of the ketogenic diet. With the flavorful and delicious recipes found in this step by step keto cookbook, they will be useful additions for any keto dieter at any stage of their ketogenic journey. I have yet to see anyone complain about having too many easy yet delicious recipes!

ONE LAST THING...

If you enjoyed this book or found it useful, I'd be very grateful if you'd post a short review on Amazon. Your support really does make a difference, and I read all the reviews personally so I can get your feedback and make this book even better.

Thanks again for your support!

Printed in Great Britain
by Amazon

76450523R10066